AF256714

Abortion
(or Woman as Threefold Murderess)

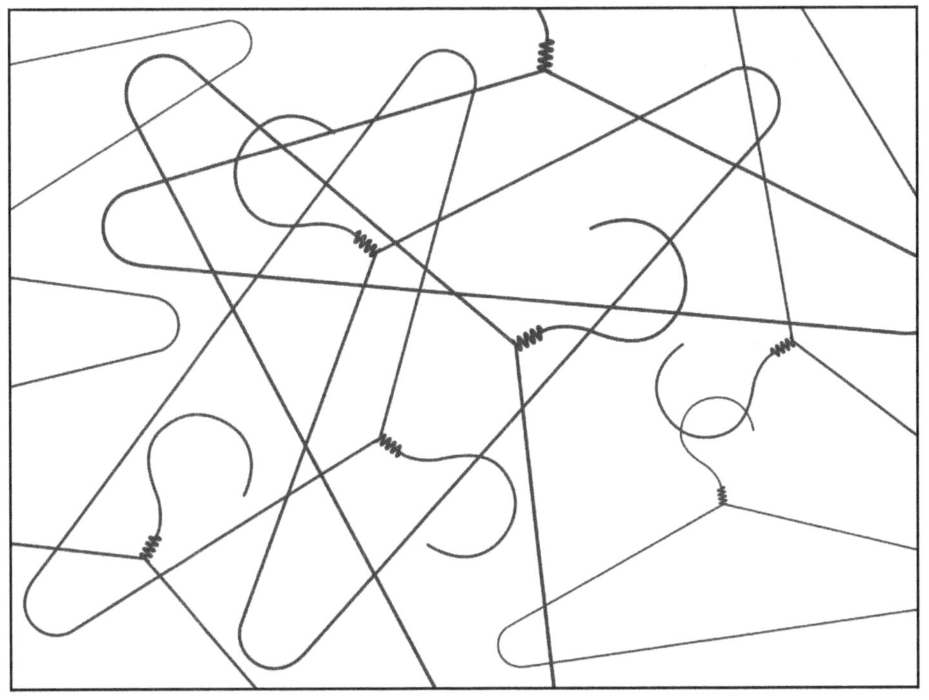

Judy Juanita

EquiDistance Press
Oakland

The threefold murderess is a term that comes from antiquity. Human reproductive scientist D. Malcolm Potts of UC Berkeley said St. Jerome (c. 342–347 to 420) was particularly uncharitable in describing women who died from attempting an abortion as a "threefold murderess: as suicides, as adulteress to their heavenly bridegroom Christ and as murderess of their still unborn child."

found poem/haiku from my mother Marguerite Juanita Hart

> *all my babies*
> *were diaphragm*
> *babies*

Abortion (or Woman as Threefold Murderess)

A compendium on abortion, date rape, parenting, and adoption in four genres: nonfiction, short stories, poetry, and testimonies, written and compiled by Judy Juanita

ISBN: 978-1-7326098-1-5

The anonymous testimonies in "Testimonies from Women with Multiple Abortions" come from the Shout Your Abortion website:

https://shoutyourabortion.com/stories/

"The Long History of Abortion" factoids come from two sources:

Malcolm Potts — Potts, M. et al. "Thousand-year-old depictions of massage abortion," Journal of Family Planning and Reproductive Health Care, volume 33, page 234 (2007)"

CC BY-SA 3.0, https://commons.wikimedia.org/w/index.php?curid=6300604; https://www.glowm.com/section-view/item/375

Jahdeen Brown lives in Oakland but was born and raised in Jamaica. He wrote his poem in a creative writing class at Laney College in response to the poem "the powerful nurse, the powerful baby." He has an A.A. degree from Laney College and a B.A. degree from SFSU.

not, if the performance is public or private; for charity or gain. This excludes classroom use and auditions which the author encourages. For performance of any part of this copyrighted work or the whole — at "readings" as well as "performances" — please seek licensing fee information from:

Equidistance Press
490 Lake Park Ave
P.O. Box 16053
Oakland, CA 94610
whoknewyouknew@gmail.com
www.judyjuanita.com

Preface

Abortion is at the forefront of issues facing our tumultuous society. Physicians in Texas cannot even broach the subject to women facing life-threatening miscarriages; they're letting the women go into sepsis rather than help them and face criminal charges themselves. Recently a friend and mother of two grown children told me that she aborted her third pregnancy at six months. She hadn't wanted more children nor had her husband and thus decided to abort. I didn't hear more of what she said—details which I normally am attuned to—because I was shocked and upset. The fetus is generally thought to be viable at 24 weeks or six months in. Had my friend murdered her child? Was this an immoral act? How different was her decision in her 30s or 40s from my decision at 21 years old with two fewer months than her pregnancy? I thought at 21 and for years afterwards that many people wouldn't have approved of my decision to abort in the second trimester. I didn't discuss it out loud. My fiancé knew that it was probably not his; we married two months later and brought our child into life 14 months later.

I will not set myself up as my friend's conscience nor be another adult's ethical guide, even though I know many laws attempt to do just that. My position remains that (1) it's a woman's right to choose, and (2) proper medical care should be available to all women as they traverse the difficult journey of deciding to bear a child. How far into the pregnancy they should be able to abort remains a jurisdictional issue, not a ministerial decision, a public health issue, not a political football, pending a national constitutional amendment. My writing examines the misguided idea that choosing to abort is an easy decision. Rather, I try to show that unilaterally it's an uneasy decision, using memoir, narrative nonfiction, personal narrative, and narrative journalism.

I look at the circumstances surrounding my abortion some decades back when I was a young, vulnerable college militant in the 1960s in the midst of political and sexual revolution. I was a recipient of The California Therapeutic Abortion Act passed in June, 1967. I posit that my abortion was an act of violence during an era of violence in a violence-driven society. My abortion, in April 1968, left an ugly scar on my psyche, nothing on my body which probably helped submerge it for so long.

Much personal truth in my life has evolved from large social movements: my parents' migration from Oklahoma to California, growing up in the black church, my time in the Black Panther Party and the Black student movement, my Buddhist faith, all big communal waves. I've experienced each in an intensely personal way. As a member of the first Black Student Union in the nation at SF State, I was tasked with finding an apartment for then-visiting lecturer LeRoi Jones and his pregnant wife Sylvia.[1] I failed to find them a rental (and was forever mortified), despite walking all around Fillmore-Haight with $250 of school monies in my purse. He had left a white wife, two mixed babies, and bohemia in Greenwich Village to jumpstart the Black Nationalist movement first in Harlem, then in Newark. We heard through the grapevine that in New Jersey he had in rapid order impregnated a young black woman Olabumi and fallen in love with Sylvia.[2] Olabumi was to die suddenly and the fated lovers tainted by the double death of mother and baby-in-utero, so romantic and so tragic. It was clear to me that ruptured love was a necessary feature of The Revolution. Her blooming belly at his readings signified all that The Movement meant. Follow your man and the cause through hell and high water.

This book took six decades to break through my blackout (pun intended). Nevertheless, in my fiction, poetry, and drama, pregnant or aborting women or aborted babies keep showing up, like unannounced house guests. I've included a set of my short stories that are abortion-themed and a few poems, also abortion-themed. Finally, two appendices give an abbreviated history of abortion techniques since antiquity and biblical times up through the legalization of abortion (Appendix I) and, more recently, anonymous testimonies of women who have had multiple abortions (Appendix II).

---

[1] They would go on to become Amiri Baraka and Amina Baraka
[2] Baraka's *The Autobiography of LeRoi Jones* (1984, 2012) details what was rumored to my crew in 1969

We need to thrash out choice long and hard, even with the overturning of Roe v. Wade[3], the same way that we are grappling with health/sexuality/food and drug regulation, immigration, gun control, and other matters. I am pro-choice but would love this deafeningly loud, necessary debate to allow a much greater measure of sensitivity and nuance.

— Judy Juanita
Oakland, CA
October, 2025

---

[3]Landmark Supreme Court ruling that established a woman's constitutional right to an abortion, based on the right to privacy under the Fourteenth Amendment. The 7–2 decision determined that states could not ban abortions, particularly in the first three months of pregnancy, but established a trimester framework where the state's interest in protecting fetal life increased with the progress of the pregnancy. This ruling, however, was overturned in 2022 by the Supreme Court in the Dobbs v. Jackson Women's Health Organization case, effectively ending the federal right to abortion and returning regulatory power to individual states.

Foreword

As a licensed clinical psychologist, I have had the honor of working with many women and families who faced the choice to have an abortion (and yes, young girls who had the choice of conception taken from them by perpetrators who forced their will upon them). Some of those individuals chose to keep their baby, a choice that sometimes led to tremendous joy at choosing parenthood and other times led to resentment towards the child for existing.

Many people on both sides of the pro-choice/pro-life continuum erroneously believe the act of having an abortion is a simple decision, that it is always a choice and that choice is always black or white. In my experience, that is not the case. Many of the children I saw for therapy due to abuse, neglect, and trauma were the product of "pro-life" families/communities. That is not to say that some of the children I saw in similar situations were not from pro-choice families/communities, but I will say that some of the most horrific cases I worked with involved children from pro-life ideology families/communities. Regardless of the circumstances that led to the decision to terminate a pregnancy, I can say with absolute certainty that not one of the girls/women/families I worked with who had to make the choice to abort were making it as a primary option to birth control.

I saw often that the most loving thing that could be done was to terminate life prior to full gestation; I saw it often enough to leave me with the conviction that those who were terminated were deeply wanted and deeply loved. Many people I worked with who made the choice to have an abortion grappled with grief of the life that could have been, accompanied by guilt for the relief they felt for the life they had without the added hardships of parenthood. Not once did a person leave my office "happy" about choosing to end a life regardless of the circumstances.

The choice to have an abortion often required a lifelong journey of healing for the individual, as did the choice not to. This is far more nuanced than anyone can truly comprehend. Healing for those faced with the decision to keep or terminate a pregnancy does not happen from chastising someone for whatever choice they will make (or made), nor does it happen from stripping access to appropriate care services, both medically and psychologically. As psychologists, our primary obligation is to protect the confidentiality of our clients, which includes providing informed care and a safe place to heal. It is to give a voice to all experiences of the human condition- including the decision to choose.

Judy Juanita has spent her life's work giving a voice to disenfranchised communities. To date, her body of work masterfully captures the nuances and complexities of human experiences in various facets such as race, gender, higher education, socioeconomic status, and political revolutions. In this book, she extends that body of work to include various phases of parental choice. While the title might suggest this is a book condemning the choice of abortion, it is in fact the opposite- and on a side note, anyone who has had the privilege of meeting/knowing Judy knows she would never condemn anyone for any choice they made (or did not make).

Reading *Abortion (or Woman as Threefold Murderess)*, I felt like I was sitting in therapy sessions with any number of my clients while they recounted touchstone events that forever shaped their lives. The essays and short stories provide snapshots into the psychological complexities of choosing to keep a pregnancy or have an abortion, highlighting the impact each choice may have on future life templates. The real gem of this book is the vulnerability and authenticity captured by the stories, testimonies, and poems, in a way that could have only been done by someone who has the utmost love and care for life.

—Dr. Marita Padilla, PsyD, ABPP
Licensed Clinical Psychologist

Table of contents

"the powerful nurse, the powerful baby" • "It's ok Mommy"
• "I love hospitals. Loved them since I was a girl" • "The
philosopher"

"Glimpses of the Long History of Abortion" •
"Ways to Abort or Prevent Pregnancy, 19th century
onward" • "Woman as Threefold Murderess" • "An
abortion practice in a Welsh mining community
in the 1920s" • "Plants used as abortifacients and
emmenagogues by Spanish New Mexicans" •

"1959"

Genre: Essay

"Deciding on Womanhood"

Over and over, when she pressed and braided my hair, my mother told me the story of her older sister's abortion. My nine year old mind, simply fascinated, took it all in, the cautionary tale, the blood, gore, and secrecy. Auntie had been a fast gal — but brainy as all get out — in small town Oklahoma. She went away to college on scholarship and came home on break pregnant. Grandmother proceeded to set up an old-fashioned home abortion. My mother witnessed it all and, in her inimitable way, fed me the gory details. Getting your hair pressed with a hot comb means sitting as still as possible to avoid the dreaded ear nick from that hot iron. But I sat patiently hoping not to get burned and waiting for the upbeat ending. The big sister returned to college, went on to an illustrious career as a librarian, became a prominent soror, respectable wife and mother, and esteemed member of the black middle class. She lived to 94 and Mom to 92. My mother and father migrated to California in the 1940s and birthed four of us, a book in itself.

Back in time, however, back in Oklahoma, my mother had set off for the black college, Langston University, and in her first semester was date-raped. She, too, became pregnant. Her outcome was different. Having seen an actual abortion, she wanted none of it. She defied Grandmother and refused to abort. That story "Hometown Buffet" is in the short story collection, *The High Price of Freeways,* and included in this book. Mom practically dictated it to me near the end of her life. My brother and I had heard about this phantom first baby but never the particulars. That's the way family secrets unfold, bit by bit.

Around that time in Oklahoma, during The Great Depression, a set of triplets began the journey to adoption and separation. A new mouth to feed was frightening enough during the Depression, multiple births catastrophic. My mother told me the story of the girls' births. The sister of her best friend from college adopted two of the girls. Families often "farmed out" twins, triplets or quadruplets. "Triplets" in this collection about abortion, birthing, and parenting presents one more utilitarian solution to unwanted childbirth.

In 2019, I pursued my genetic results, i.e. ancestry. I swabbed, mailed the data, waited weeks, expecting to see I was part-Indian, as family lore went, and mostly African. The results showed 1.1% Indigenous

American (what!!!???); 74.7% Sub-Saharan African (expected); and 22.8% European (Pullease!). The philosopher Cornel West said these negligible amounts of Native-American blood in these ancestry tests shouldn't be surprising because, and I paraphrase him, it wasn't the Indian in the kitchen raping our grandmas, it was the Irishman. My great-grandfather was Irish. I didn't pursue any more with that.

But people pursued me from that test. One person even called my brother, and, sure enough, established that she was the daughter of my mother's long-ago given-up-for-adoption baby. That baby had loving parents and grew to become a successful adult. The past in my face! Like the ancestry report, I was too through with it, but not my brother. He and his new found kinfolk began communicating copiously. I suggested he forward her a copy of "Hometown Buffet" to see if it matched her story. It did, down to dates and everything.

Why do I tell this now? Martin Luther King said that "the arc of the moral universe is long, but it bends toward justice." The moral universe of a single abortion impacts more than the mother and unborn. I witnessed the arc of my mother's decision and her sister's decision. One didn't abort, the other did. It took decades, more than five, for me to see how each decision (and mine) played out.

"Alameda County Welfare Dept."

It was spring, 1965. I had completed two years at community college and worked fulltime at the welfare department at 401 Broadway in Oakland, in the Dictaphone transcriptionist pool, while applying to SF State. Our attitude transcribing our tapes from intake workers interviewing welfare recipients was one of ridicule. They were performers, both the social workers and the clients. We laughed at their exploits. Coming from a two-parent household with a mother who was a forty-years-and-a-gold watch civil servant, I was ignorant about welfare clients holding on economically with the life preserver of Aid to Families with Dependent Children (AFDC).

"Davita"

Davita often gave me a ride home from 401; she was married to a suave, sharp dresser named Marcus. Their union came to an abrupt end when Davita insisted on keeping a second unplanned pregnancy. She carried to term in defiance of his wishes. I heard her side every day on the ride home. But, exercising his body politic, he left her. She was in control, i.e. until he left her and both kids high and dry. I saw her power evaporate in a day. It stunned her and me. How could he leave his children? Why did she insist on a second that he didn't want? I pondered their dilemma for years.

"Audrey"

My cubicle partner at 401 was Audrey. The months that we worked together, two young black idealistic women, we read out loud William Goldman's *Boys and Girls Together* to the amusement of the other transcriptionists. I kept applying to SF State secret from everyone in the pool except Audrey. She had a secret too. She waited until my last day to tell me what it was. The pool threw a party for me, wishing me well as I set off for State. And finally, Audrey told me her secret — she had a son out of wedlock. She thought I would judge her because I had ridiculed the recipients. I was very ashamed that she thought I would think badly of her. Nevertheless I was eager to leave 401, where I saw civil servants looking forward to retiring in 15 or 20 years. I didn't want their future. Nor did I want to end up like Audrey or any of the clients on our Dictaphone tapes.

"Alone and Singing in the Opera House"

My first semester at San Francisco State, spring '66, was like a preliminary bout before the main fight. I rode across the Bay Bridge with fellow students from East Oakland that had attended State since high school. Their talk of parties, sororities, and fraternities, the black Greeks, didn't interest me at all. I wasn't a bourgie. I wasn't a snob. I had no wish to be a girlfriend of either. What I loved to do was catch the M streetcar into downtown after my classes, eat at Zim's at Market and Van Ness, then walk a few blocks to the War Memorial Opera House with its huge, empty atrium. The lobby acoustics were so awe-inspiring that I'd sing my butt off for 45 minutes, my contralto like a stag horn fern in there, in transition between ancient and modern ferns. Maybe I missed my church choir rehearsals. When I switched to soprano, I was more like a maiden hair fern. Either way passersby didn't mind. In that atrium, I felt far away from judgment.

"The Splintering of the Monolith"

I had thought of black people as one, maybe even a monolith, though I wouldn't have used that word. I had the picture in my mind, though, of all of us being outraged, despairing, and hurt by the hosing of the children in Birmingham. Yet day after day, hearing the speakers on their soapboxes in the campus common, I was honestly bewildered by the sharp divisions in the movements. All of the revolutionary groups, the Panthers, the Nation of Islam, RAM (Revolutionary Action Movement), and the black arts poets, put down the Southern Christian Leadership Conference (SCLC), Congress of Racial Equality (CORE), National Association for the Advancement of Colored People (NAACP), and the URBAN LEAGUE as accommodationist. I heard Martin Luther King scornfully called Martin Luther Queen. The Greeks, i.e. Alphas, Kappas, Omegas, Deltas, AKAs, were dismissed as passé and bourgeois. When I went to meetings or rallies off campus, I witnessed different black guys, often in daishikis or combat fatigues, trash each other. Che Guevara with his cold-blooded executioner's rep was the model. I didn't know what to think except to be glad that, with my au natural, nobody was attacking me. I felt like a fly on the wall trying not to get smashed. I joined the Black Students Union (BSU) that semester as it changed its name from the Negro Students Association. I really settled in my second full semester in fall of '66. A contingent of State students had gone down South to desegregate interstate buses, joining The Freedom Riders. When they returned, they radicalized the entire campus, students and faculty, practically everybody. I joined the Tutorial Program and almost instantaneously took charge of a Tutorial Center on Potrero Hill.

"Bernadine"

At State, I infrequently ran into Bernadine, a pretty, light-skinned probation officer whose two kids I baby sat in high school. 32 and attending San Francisco State part time, she was a divorcee who dated a lot. My street wise father, who picked me up from her house on Sunday mornings so I could go to church, thought she was scandalous. Over her fireplace was her portrait, a Bernadine pre-beating; her ex-husband had beaten her with the spoken intent to destroy her beauty and sexual allure. She'd required hospitalization. Regardless of my father's disapproval, I admired her for retaining her allure and moxie despite the scars. She was neither a bourgie nor a militant; just a single mom earning her M.A. semester-by-semester. Her tenacity showed me that keeping one's mojo took fearlessness and disregard of other's disapproval.

"Marianna"

There was also another 32 year old at San Francisco State that I observed carefully, and this 32 year old woman was an outspoken black militant who led the BSU's name change. Her sexual liaison with a younger male student from Sacramento was the scandal of the black crowd the day he came to school with a Mohawk-long before Mohawks were popular. It was said that she had convinced him to shave his head.

SF State, with its 19,000 students, mostly commuters, was a big, cosmopolitan student body that spilled across the conventional age categories of 18-22 year olds. State pulled in wayfarers from all over the U.S. and the world and all age groups, as I discovered working in the admissions office. Marianna had come up from Los Angeles, her mother a prominent sculptor and painter, to make her own way, she told me, with only a blender and a box of books. She loved my groovy earrings from a little shop on Ashby in Berkeley called "Someplace." so I turned into her procurer of earrings, 3 pairs/$10. She was like a big, robust peony, showing off the power of sex.

"Grace"

There were timid black girls there, too, like Grace, a good Catholic school girl from a family of nine children. She told everyone that she'd wanted to be a nun. She was like a delicate and brittle-stemmed sweet pea, much too vulnerable for the intense sexual politics in the BSU as well any of the Greeks. Yet, there she was, falling for one of the top dawgs (as our crew liked to call it), functioning as if she were a concubine of one of the brothers leading the movement, who conveniently put her up in an apartment next to his other girlfriend, with BSU monies, of course. It was all part of gaming or, rather, controlling, the system. We were all caught up in the thick of it, the sexual merry-go-round.

"Cecil B. DeMille"

Bennett, the film major from Milwaukee, hung around the commons, always there when I grabbed lunch, his half-compliments like fireflies. I had a mercurial attraction. Out of horniness, I considered giving him the key to the flesh-palace. He came from somewhere beside California and had aspiration, which placed him a step beyond instinct.

"I want to be the black Cecil B. DeMille," he said one afternoon.

"And direct a cast of thousands?" I shot back.

"That's right," he said. "Our story has never been told."

I corrected him. "Our stories have never been told."

He stopped as if I had placed a red light before him. "Stories… yeah, we've got lots."

"Plenty," *Cecil*. I saw Bennett, black beret on, gentleman's cravat concealing his bony shoulder blades, directing thousands of black extras streaming around the Lincoln Memorial, the only place I'd ever seen thousands of blacks. He interrupted my dream.

"I want to shoot you," he said.

"Shoot me? Why? What did I do to you?"

"You know, take a lot of pictures," he shrugged. "Clothes on, clothes off."

"You want nudie pictures of me?"

"It's art. Art and nudity go hand in hand."

"And where would your hand go?" The mercury dropped, the door to the palace closed. Boom. Shut. He looked sheepish, not Cecil B. DeMille-ish.

"Charlotte"

Charlotte at 16 years old began hanging around the BSU office and the Party. With her bright smile, devotion to task, Catholic school blue serge uniform and white knee socks, she proceeded to run through a host of brothers. Years later, she would become a Muslim and wear a hijab resolutely covering everything except that smile. I could sense a penitence in the beautiful folds of her long robes. When I mentioned recently to one of the Central Committee that technically the brothers basically ran a train on her and were risking statutory rape, I got cussed out.

"Violence an Overpowering Norm"

Violence was an overpowering norm in the world with Viet Nam raging in Southeast Asia and the civil rights movement raging in the South. I began perceiving violence as a norm in the smaller world surrounding me. I tried to dodge the verbal gunfire. How could I speak scathingly of my family, church people from my childhood, even my girlfriends from high school? I tried it one time. My dad and I met up at a store, ironically called White Front in East Oakland. I repeated the rhetoric I'd heard on campus, that Negroes like him were going to end up in concentration camps because of their passivity to "the man" — the catchall term for the white man's system. Nothing could have been further from the reality of my dad's life. He had been a "race man" down South, i.e. a black man who wouldn't tolerate oppression. When he was a Tuskegee Airman in WWII, he had protested the restrictive seating in downtown Tuskegee, Alabama theaters before his regiment shipped to Italy. But I was in full rebel mode, daring to sass him with the linguistic violence that had become my daily diet.

Cutting ties to our parents, the institutions of our childhood, mainly the black church, was de rigueur. One of my roomies, who called herself a black militant, returned to Third Baptist Church, San Francisco's oldest African-American church, to sing every Sunday in the choir. She was ridiculed for going but her tie remained unbroken for the rest of her life.

Nutritional violence came from the Nation of Islam. Cut your addiction to pork was the mantra. To be seen eating bacon or a ham sandwich in the school cafeteria was tantamount to being a fool. Muslims in bowties and suits surrounded the table and castigated the black students (not the whites) eating lunch. I gave up my beloved grilled ham and cheese for The Movement.

This concept of slash, give up, turn from, do away with was across the board. Physical. Emotional. Religious. Interpersonal. Linguistic violence came in the slogans and sloganeering, *Off the Pig*, *Black Power to Black People*, and the great ethnic change from *colored people* and *Negro* to *Black* to *African-American*. Heaven help the poor pitiful person who slipped and used the wrong term in the wrong place. But because people are only human, not everyone could live up to the strict revolutionary codes. Thus, deceits, treachery, and manipulation were part of The Movement. *Black is beautiful* was another mantra that holds to this day. My roomie asked me not to tell anyone that she used Nadinola, a skin bleaching cream I had stumbled on in her toiletries. Women who fell in love with or chose brothers who were cultural nationalists wore long dresses and elaborate African head wraps. Someone sat me down and explained that in a riot or at a protest, when the cops started swinging, I'd better be able to run fast. Ergo, jeans were feasible, not long skirts. I cut up my jeans and wore torn tee shirts, an act of wardrobe violence.

And it's not as though the women were relegated to childbearing and cooking. Kathleen Cleaver, Elaine Brown, Angela Davis, and the black women poets of the era were just as staccato and bristling as the pork-denying Muslims.

"Sonia Sanchez"

Sonia was yet another force for change. A tiny high-strung woman in her early 30s, her poetry was forceful, militant, strident, utterly sensual. My roomies and I emulated her, hung out with her, even babysat her children until she abruptly left San Francisco amidst a romance gone sour. Sonia Sanchez commented recently on the her work in that era: "You must remember, in the time that we were writing, all the death and dying that happened and how we had discovered how much we'd been enslaved in this country… We came out hitting and slapping and alerting people to what had happened" (*The Writer's Chronicle*, Feb. 2014:29).

"Gwendolyn Brooks"

Gwendolyn Brooks, a gentler, 50 year old Pulitzer Prize winning poet, spent time on campus too, accompanying the much younger poet Don L. Lee. They carried themselves like lovers. They sat *thisclose* like lovers. It was clear she was his mentor, but to my eyes and to my roomies they were a May-December romance. She had left her long marriage and would soon break with her mainstream New York publisher Harper's and embrace black cultural nationalism. Don Lee became Haki Madhubuti and his Third World Press her publisher. It was a time of dramatic change for blacks and the entire country… and me.

"Deciding on Activism"

Bobby Seale and Huey Newton came to San Francisco State in spring, '67 to recruit at the same time Clorox, Kaiser and IBM came. The two men stood side by side, gave their spiel, their sign-up sheets laid out in the back of the room. My roommates and I, our hair au natural, in pea coats, ponchos and boots, listened. I knew the two men from community college. But I hesitated when my buddies signed to join the Black Panther Party (BPP), remembering my civil servant mother's warning about signing my name to radical causes — *never sign away your name, your body or your birthright*. While some came to call it the Summer of Love, for those of us in the belly of the beast — urban America, it was another long, hot summer. By August, I joined. On October 28, Huey and the Oakland PD got into it. One officer died; Huey was shot and charged with charged with murder and assault. The BPP goes into its next evolution, Free Huey, the campaign that Eldridge creates. It's as bloody and violent as childbirth, and I'm in the middle of it.

"Five Young Women"

We five — Janice, Jo Ann, Betty, Evelyn and I — became the first wave of students from State to join the Party. Evelyn handled party finances; Betty managed the office; Janice was Bobby's scheduler, Jo Ann corralled the troops, and I worked on the newspaper. We remain enrolled but spend our waking hours with the BPP in the office and the community. Our nine-room flat on Potomac St overlooking Duboce Park, which had been(unbeknownst to us) Alcoholics Anonymous' first meeting place, would turn into a BPP safe house. Our gang of five formed romantic and sexual liaisons from the upper echelon to the lumpen proletariat. The BSU brothers like to talk about supplying the BPP with guns and money, but *this bridge called my back* supplied the people's army with equal and greater provision.

"Huey Appoints Me Editor-in-Chief"

After Huey was jailed in the shootout in November 1967, the paper overnight became an international organ, and the party the radical arm of the civil rights movement. From jail, Huey appointed me editor-in-chief, transforming my life instantly. The Panthers created what Jean-Paul Sartre calls superlanguage, i.e. the colonized deconstruct their oppression and make the language revolutionary, incantatory: *Off the pigs. Power to the people. Free Huey.* The iconic representations focused on men strapped with bandoliers and guns and the marches and protests (hard power) v. Women/Men in the community service programs (soft power). Yet, two-thirds to seventy percent of the BPP was female.

"Assassination"

Martin Luther King Jr. was assassinated on Thursday, April 4th, 1968. Riots broke out across the nation. D.C., Baltimore, Chicago, and Kansas City erupted in flames. The night of the West Oakland shoot-out, my boyfriend Buzz, a party member and fellow State student, and I had decided to get married. We visit his Uncle Ike on Saturday, April 6, to tell him and his wife about the engagement and wedding in two months. Ike had been Eldridge's probation officer, and Eldridge had mentioned Ike in *Soul on Ice.* We hear about the shootout on the way home on the radio. In minutes, we find out that Lil' Bobby Hutton, the first recruit to join the party, was gunned down on Saturday, April 6th. A 39-year-old activist pastor in Memphis, and a 17-year-old activist in Oakland. The unbelievable keeps happening.

The next day, after the shootout, Buzz and I had gone out to eat and come back to my little apartment at 1518 Julia St. in Berkeley. It looked like someone had broken in through the front window of the apartment. Inside were Bobby, Jo Ann, Evelyn, Janice, and the white couple Alex and Elsa Knight Thompson — he was a Party lawyer and she was the broadcaster from KPFA, the Pacifica radio station. They explained to us that we were all on the run from the police.

All I could see was my dirty laundry and my underwear, spilled all over the living room floor. I was beyond embarrassed, but Bobby said, 'We've got to go.' For the rest of that night, Bobby, Jo Ann, Evelyn, Janice, Buzz, and I eluded the police, the FBI, assassins, agent provocateurs, who knows, running through backyards in West Oakland and South Berkeley. Alex and Elsa kept up for half the time before they took refuge along the chase. We were amazed at how limber Bobby was. He was the oldest, but he jumped those fences like a teenager. Bobby said that Huey was adamant that Oakland not go down in flames — "no spontaneous riots." We finally made it to a safe apartment. Stokeley said black people are good at revolts, but revolution requires a lifetime of determined activity. Oakland was not going to have a riot after these horrendous events! As we let down our guard and got food from the kitchen of the apartment, Bobby said to me and Buzz, "You guys wanna fuck, you can use the bedroom." I could only think that fucking was the very last thing on my mind.

We returned to campus that fall, armed with a new consciousness that birthed the longest student strike in American history and changed the face of American higher education.

"Kathleen Cleaver"

We meet up, the roomies and I, on the landing of the admin building
at State. We just got married, Eldridge tells us, pride of ownership all
over his face. She comes off shy like a bride but coiled like a panther;
she is high yellow, green-eyed, with a puffed brown sugar natural,
black boots and turtleneck, wired for takeoff. The green eyes speak to
us. They say: get back. She extends a smile. I hear him say: she was
George Ware's secretary. I can't see her taking care of nobody's stuff.
That's what we're here for.

"Agent Provocateurs???"

These two guys from SNCC in LA—or who said they were from
SNCC in LA, visited the BSU offices at State, ultra-cool, ultra-blasé
revolutionaries wearing the hell out of their regulation overalls and
denim jackets I had been busy getting my paycheck, didn't have time
to listen to their rap. I was trying to get paid not laid. When I got back
from the bank, they were still holding court. The large one was vocif-
erous, the quiet one smiled at what was being said. I thought they were
talking about organizing the South, maybe the ultimate cattle prod
story, judging from how captivated people looked. But the big guy was
going on about sex as calmly as if he was recommending vaccination.
"Mothers should give their young sons head and fathers should initiate
young daughters into the mysteries of oral copulation." I couldn't
believe my ears.

People looked disgusted and walked out. I don't know why I stayed, I
didn't agree with him. "Parents have to show their children the way of
the world. A parent can do it gently, wisely, slowly." He used his hands
graphically. More people walked. "This is too important to leave to
chance or strangers" It made sense, but it didn't make sense. The two
of them looked, talked, walked, and moved like movement people but
maybe they weren't. Maybe they were agents. Maybe they were evil.

Once I joined the BPP, they taught us that agents and agent-provocateurs always proposed the most extreme, most outlandish action, more derring-do than deliberate. At the moment it intrigued me.

"The Free Breakfast for Children Program"

The core of the party's Survival Programs was a community service program that provided a free breakfast before school. The Party launched it in January 1969 at St. Augustine's Episcopal Church in Oakland, Father Earl Neil's church. A church member, Ruth Beckford-Smith, the Bay Area's premiere interpreter of modern African dance, was in charge of this first program. It had sprung from the vision of Huey and Bobby, inspired by the belief that alleviating hunger and poverty was necessary for Black liberation and by the essential role of breakfast for learning. The program was a direct response to the war on poverty in the 60s, the U.S. government's promise to provide basic needs (housing, food, safety) to its citizens. Ruth Beckford and Father Neil constructed a healthy menu and a kitchen and dining hall that passed health inspections. The program's launch day served 11 children. By the end of the week 135 children were being served daily. Volunteers set up around 6 am and served the meal from 7 — 8:30. Everybody pitched in, no matter our other duties.

"The first martyr Lil Bobby"

I cry picturing Lil Bobby, scared in the basement, refusing to take off his clothes to save his ass, prison-savvy Eldridge stripping naked, emerging into the lethal spotlight. The peacock lived, the peachick died. The brothers in P.E. class who were there talk of a volley of bullets electrifying Lil Bobby. Lynching up north. The panthers wore indigo and black; the cops wore indigo and black, a brotherhood of measure.

"Lumpen proletariat shit"

I shoplift a boatload of shit, books, records, clothes, scarves, grades. I get quite good at it, a master, the good girl-turned-slippery eel until I got caught. My shoplifting case gets postponed for several months, at my repeated requests, hoping the BPP would come to my rescue magically. They're fighting big battles, political battles, life and death battles. But Bobby Seale sits me down, listens to my story and tells me about a 50-foot area outside the store. If I was arrested inside the area, which I was, I can plead not guilty on the grounds that I had forgotten to pay. Bobby instructs me on how to question the store manager and emphasize that he never asked if I had stolen something and didn't discuss it while we waited for the police. I feel a bit ashamed to take up his time, but Bobby handles it like it was routine.

Am I a common thief, I ask myself, when I see the lumpen proletariat in court, stammering, confessing, begging for mercy. A young man who stole a deck of cards, worth less than a dollar — 30 days in Santa Rita County Jail; a young white woman who confessed to stealing a $5 bathing suit from Woolworth's — six months on the prison farm; a black man who burglarised, a white girl who left the scene of an accident, a Latino youth who stole petty cash from an employer — jail, jail, jail. I am petrified; everybody is getting time. The courtroom clears out, leaving the prosecutor, store manager, judge, court reporter, all white, and me. Using Bobby's strategy and my best collegiate voice I take the stand. The judge allows me to ask questions of the manager who can't remember what he asked me outside the store. He didn't know how many feet I had gone before being stopped. I get the feeling that he had expected a repeat of the past two hours — stammering hasty inarticulate confessions.

My thoughts flow in two streams. In my pounding heart, I want to confess everything. But I don't want to end up under the jail. Instead I talk school, grades, reading, wanting to teach, making an honest mistake, forgetting what I'd picked up in the store until after I'd been stopped outside. The judge smiles as if lulled by either the late afternoon or my Future Teachers of America voice. He reduces the charge to malicious mischief, a misdemeanour, and fines me $25. I walk out, relieved to be free.

"Deciding on Abortion"

By 1968, I am a senior at San Francisco State when I have to see about my period. I see the people at Planned Parenthood. I am so busy on deadline for the Black Panther Party intercommunal newspaper and working part-time at UCSF Medical Center that I forget to go back for the results. Between visits I tell my roomie. I know she has a sympathetic mind. And that's what I need, not someone to tell me what to do.

I ask her to go horseback riding with me on Skyline Blvd. in Oakland. Horseback riding was one of the classy dates, classy that is at the start of an affair. But if you got pregnant, so I heard, horseback riding dislodged the fetus, made you abort. We go early the next day. I ride my horse at a gallop, enough to bounce up and down, enough to bring a period down. It hurts but I have to do it. She rides her horse like a mule, poking along. No blood. Planned Parenthood (PP) closes on the weekend.

I can't wait for a yes or a no. She watches as I take Carter's little liver pills by the tens. Maybe I can get sick and have my stomach pumped. I have never been sick. I don't know anything but good health. I take 100 Carter's little liver pills. I feel a slight nausea, nothing more than I've felt on and off for weeks. I don't go to the hospital. I don't get pumped. I show up at PP bright and early. They give it to me, the dim late words: you're expecting. No, don't tell me I'm pregnant. I only screwed once in this whole time period. The dr says: "It's the Immaculate Conception, we hear about it all the time."

The next two weeks are frantic. I know I'm pregnant, no one else knows. If I don't tell anyone, then no one else ever has to know. I gather options:

- leave the country and have an abortion in Norway (this from a doctor to a student);

- keep doing bodily damage until I either abort or kill myself;

- drink quinine;

- get the coat hanger.

I'm afraid. I can't hurt myself anymore. A woman at the PP said I could have crippled myself with the liver pills. She gives me a number to call. I'm afraid. Maybe she's the FBI, trying to get me to commit suicide. Maybe she's not the FBI but has contacts with abortionists, dirty-fingered men in bare-light-bulb offices. I'm afraid. I'm out of money. I go back up to UCSF Med Center to get my severance check.

When Jennifer, the 9th floor switchboard operator, greets me like old times, she thanks me for giving her my dress. (I didn't give her anything, I left it there, the RNs must have given it to her). But she is happy to see me, says, you were so different, it's so dull now. She looks at me closely, says, you look worried, what's wrong? I start to tell her and hear my voice waver; she's the first person in the City besides my roomies to show concern for me. She pulls out a memo.

It explains a new law in California permitting abortion to be legal and performed by doctors in hospitals. She gives me a number to call. It's an abortion shrink. She says, you have to visit him twice, talk with him. I frown. She says, it's more a formality… but when you go, especially the second visit, talk like it's already driving you nuts, being pregnant… act a little crazy or paranoid or something like that… then he can sign and you can get it done at Kaiser.

I end up, nearly three months along, sitting in his office in Berkeley, talking as nutty and paranoid as I can. I tell him about the sirens in San Francisco; about the FBI outside my apartment; about the teacher from high school who showed us his photos of the dead swallowed man and the man cut in half by the train, how only recently they have turned back up in my dreams; I tell him about all the agent provocateurs in the Party who make my skin crawl; I tell him about my fears. I don't have to exaggerate.

I ask him, is this enough? He nods and signs the second trimester abortion form and walks me out of the reception area. I see through the reflection in the windows the shrink standing, gaping. I don't know if it's what I told him or that he's seeing an actual live Panther.

In June 1967, the California Legislature passed the Therapeutic Abortion Act, California becoming the third state in the country after North Carolina and Colorado to legalize abortions. An estimated 18,000 illegal abortions occur annually in California, and illegal abortions are a major factor in maternal deaths. While women with money, i.e. middle-class, can get foreign or safe non-hospital abortions, poor women perform self-induced abortions or leave the task to unlicensed helpers. Nearly 80 percent of all abortion deaths occur among non-Caucasian women.

I am in the middle of my second trimester when Kaiser admits me. The California Abortion Act has a 20 week limitation from the time of conception after which a therapeutic abortion may not be given for any reason. My parents, alerted by my use of their health coverage, come to see me, disapproving but loving.

Finally, I head away from death. My abortion, the violent disposal of an unwanted baby, will change my feelings forever about sex and sexuality. Carefree and careless become careful and cautious. But, for the now, I barely take a day off from my pressing revolutionary duties at the newspaper. Such is the life of a twenty-one year-old black activist/movement worker in Oakland in 1968. Echoing in my ear is the refrain I put in a headline for the BPP newspaper from H. Rap Brown, "Violence is as American as cherry pie."

Emory, the BPP's artist, and I put the paper together; he shows me how to hand-letter headlines, pressing out Instatype; cut and paste, we work at ease; kind and talented, his absolute devotion to the party guides what we do; we do it all, it seems. Emory and Matilaba do all the artwork, I type anything handwritten that needs to go to the typesetters, and I assist with the layout. Huey, Bobby, Eldridge give us items; speeches, addresses, position papers. Huey and Eldridge write prolifically from jail. We use solicited articles, telegrams from the famous and notable, poetry, rally news, announcements, quotes from the pantheon at will — Mao, Fanon, Marx, Che. I proudly layout a Western Union telegram from Betty Shabazz.

"Betty Shabazz"

718APST APR 12 68 LD081L 0LB088 DL PDB TOOL MTVERNON
NY 12 711A PST.

BOBBY JAMES HUTTON FAMILY, CARE KATHLEEN CLEAVERS

850 OAK St OAKLAND CALIF THE QUESTION IS NOT WILL
IT BE NON-VIOLENCE VERSUS VIOLENCE BUT WHETHER A
HUMAN BEING CAN PRACTICE HIS GOD GIVEN RIGHT OF
SELF-DEFENSE.SHOT DOWN LIKE A COMMON ANIMAL HE
DIED A WARRIOR FOR BLACK LIBERATION. IF THE GENER-
ATION BEFORE HIM HAD NOT BEEN AFRAID HE PERHAPS
WOULD BE ALIVE TODAY. REMEMBER LIKE SOLOMON
THERE IS A TIME FOR EVERYTHING. A TIME TO BE BORN, A
TIME TO DIE, A TIME TO LOVE, A TIME TO HATE, A TIME TO
FIGHT AND A TIME TO RETREAT. IN THE NAME OF BROTH-
ERHOOD AND SURVIVAL REMEMBER BOBBY. IT COULD
BE you YOUR SON YOUR HUSBAND OR YOUR BROTHER
TOMORROW. CRIMES AGAINST AN INDIVIDUAL ARE OFTEN
CRIMES AGAINST AN ENTIRE NATION. TO HIS FAMILY ONLY
TIME CAN ELIMINATE THE PAIN OF LOSING HIM BUT MAY
HE BE REMEMBERED IN THE HEARTS AND MINDS OF ALL
US.

— BETTY SHABAZZ

I feel comforted. She is mother to all that swirls around her fallen
husband's words. We take amphetamines near deadline so we can make
it. When I shit, I cannot believe the foot and a half length of my stools. I
go three days without sleep, my skin itching in spite of showers.

"Kathleen"

The roomies and I go to Eldridge's one morning, waiting for Kathleen. When she comes in the room, she has the same look she wore when we were first introduced. We see her beauty marks, the black and blue ones; this morning they're on her legs. We get the elbows to going, the eyes to rolling. Sometimes they're on her arms. Sometimes her face. I wish somebody would try to beat on me like a damn drum, I don't care how famous his ass is. This is repellent... and entertaining. We talk about it casually; everyone does.

In jail, behind the glass, Eldridge says he wishes Kathleen had an automatic beating machine so she could beat herself while he's gone. Eldridge issues an edict that brothers need to get married so they can concentrate on the Revolution (instead of pussy). The edict from Huey is to get our cars legally registered and insured to stop squandering the Defense Fund on petty car busts. We're told to get our U.S. passports in order to be able to leave the country at a moment's notice. These edicts come down through the ranks with rapidity.

"ED and Violence"

I didn't know break-and-entry as in the BSU brothers breaking into the school paper at State throwing punches at the white boys could lead to night fright (when a guy can't get it up, you know), didn't know about that until the entire central committee of the BSU, including my boyfriend, got it, performance anxiety, erectile dysfunction. They didn't know they had it either. Each one thought only he had it with one of us who was his lady or, I suppose, the second lady or for heaven's sake, the third. I thought it was my fault. He thought it was my fault. We thought it was my fault. I tried to open wider, suck smoother, talk softer until the grapevine started dropping rumoricious little grapes. One by one it turned out none of the brothers could get it up. It wasn't me. It wasn't us. It was the inexplicable working of fright. Scare the hell out of somebody else. You scare the hell out of yourself.

"The Caste System as Interpersonal Violence"

The natural hairdo formed a caste system, with "straight-haired sisters" being relegated and called out even. A poem my roomie had written and had me read often got round applause and hoots. It had a popular line belittling sisters with Vidal Sassoon haircuts and go-go boots.

Skin color was a holdover caste from centuries of mulatto privilege. The top women in the BPP, ones with visibility and prominence were Kathleen Cleaver, Ericka Huggins, Elaine Brown, Angela Davis, all light skinned.

Of the BSU brothers on the Central Committee, most had light skinned girlfriends and wives or partners lighter-skinned than themselves. In my case, my brownness contrasted with my boyfriend-then-husband who was dark-skinned.

- Alma was the wife of the second president of the Black Student Union. She was a personal friend, our commonality being our men on the BSU Central Committee. We had our first babies at the same time. She was a dynamite cook and we often cooked meals together. She and Bennie had married before he started his activist phase. She had striking shoulder-length, pressed and permed hair and wore it defiantly. The brothers were relentless in pushing her to go au natural. She adamantly refused. I proudly wore my natural but had a laissez-faire attitude about other women's hairdos. Live and let live, I thought; the advent and popularity of the natural hairdo meant that, finally, black women were freed up from the hot comb and could choose to fashion their hair as they chose. I still feel that way. One of the biggest arguments in my relationship came when my man, who loved Alma's cooking, disparaged her one evening while we were at home talking. I pointed out the hypocrisy of sitting at her table, eating her food, yet disrespecting her personhood. He scoffed at my reasoning. We went back and forth. I picked up a large glass ashtray (neither of us smoked cigarettes but lit up weed on the regular). I heaved it at him. Luckily he ducked because it hit the door and left a dent in the wood. Astounded, he said, "You're the kind of woman my father warned me about. He said a woman who can't use her fists is far more dangerous because she'll pick up something that can kill you." I was as astounded as he was at my gut violence; that I was as capable of violence as anyone else.

- Several semesters after the Black Studies Dept. had been established, most of the Central Committee brothers graduated and transitioned from being the most powerful people on a 19,000 student campus, leaders of the longest student strike in the history of American higher education, and developers of the nation's first Black Studies Department. They became regular college graduates looking for work. Several came up with a scheme for counterfeit money. My guy brought some of the bills with our household money. I thought it looked patently bogus and told him to take it around the corner to the Chinese grocer. He did, and the person behind the counter passed it back to him without saying a word. However, the FBI and the CIA were watching all of us. We were revolutionaries. The FBI got wind of the counterfeit scheme and called in the brothers one by one for interrogation. Of the bunch, only D. broke down and gave up names. One brother ended up doing time for a year. The rest of them, the Central Committee, cold-shouldered D. for snitching. Alma and I thought they were being harsh and used pillow talk for nearly a year to get them to relent. Finally they did, and D. was embraced again.

"Sexual politics or sexual boutique?"

The role of women and sexuality within revolutionary movements of the 1960s and 1970s impacted me as both participant and witness. I was a student activist and political activist in several movements, including the country's ground-breaking Black Student Union at SFSU from 1966–1972, the Black Panther Party from 1967–1969, and the nation's first Black Studies Department at SFSU from 1969–1970. Our sexual presence, acquiescence, devotion, willingness, and escapades supported each of these revolutions. Women used their sexuality and sexual relationships to support and sustain the revolutionary activities.

At San Francisco State during the revolution of the 60s, BSU brothers ran guns and women. One who set his harem up in adjacent apartments, and graced one of my roomies with his majestic virility, had the nerve to tell me, decades later after I wrote *Virgin Soul*, that my account of sexual escapades wasn't valuable to the history of the revolution of the sixties because they were secondary to the revolution. Bullshit! Our sexual devotion, escapades and all, made revolution bearable. I told another brother from the revolution about

- A pair of young sisters from Seattle attending Mills College, high yellow and high bourgie, lived in a swank apartment facing Lake Merritt. Brothers couldn't resist. They too were ran through.

- A teenage volunteer, no more than 14, high yellow and voluptuous, was snatched by Eldridge who ravished her for three days. When her mother came to the BPP office looking for her, my roomies made excuses for her disappearance and simultaneously pressured the brothers to make Eldridge return her to the office, which he did.

He was incredulous. That's why I write about it here. Future activists need to see the fuller picture. Sexual dynamics make the world go around and they make revolutions occur. Women's sexuality, childbirths and abortions, and sexual politics were integral parts of these movements. However, there were also tensions and debates around the value and role of women's sexual exploits within the movements.

In 1967, I threw my birth control pills down the toilet, in an act of rebellion against being a pawn for black male sexuality. I would wait for love with a man who wanted me exclusively. It took a while to find that kind of love.

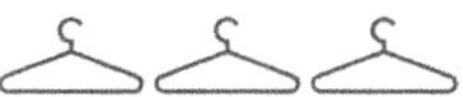

At Bread Loaf Writers Conference in 2012, I read a chapter of *Virgin Soul*, my semi-autobiographical novel documenting the black revolution that established Black Studies as a discipline. Several white women came up to me at Bread Loaf and said they went through the exact same thing in SDS (Students for a Democratic Society) and YSA (Young

Socialists Alliance). I read Che Guevara's biography, *Che Guevara: A Revolutionary life* and saw the exact same phenomenon. Why is it so hard to face that using young women and their sexual vulnerability, their adoration of the top dogs and the simultaneous oppression of them, is key to everything political?

Much time would pass before I was able to write about it, and even then fiction was the means to voice that trauma, as if my unbridled voice and witness was too much. I created a character, an alter ego, Mimi, in one story that revisited the sixties scene in retrospect:

> Mimi had felt uncomfortable the last time she had visited the Big House, as the Black Student Union had named a two-story Victorian in the Fillmore district in San Francisco. Guys were doing lines, rolling joints, watching a porno movie playing on the wall, the same brothers who had led the longest student strike in history at State and established the nation's first black studies program there, the very same brothers who had faced off the police in Hunter's Point, West Oakland and East Palo Alto, the same brothers who finagled student body funds and bought guns for the Black Panther Party, who just a decade previous had been all over sisters with naturals and averse to sisters with pressed hair. A vision of a woman's creamy white butt and pink nipples crammed the wall in the darkened room. Someone had turned off the soundtrack, so the woman's moaning and coming hard as rocks could be imagined from her mouth opening wide and her body convulsing. Miles' quintet blasted "Nefertiti" from the stereo. That was the way Mimi had learned to get high: Turn off the TV and its white noise. Keep the set on. Put Miles or Coltrane on the box and start rolling. The politics, demonstrations, rage, cries for society to explode with justice for all, had come down to this. Sex on the wall. White sex.

> "Why are brothers who're supposed to be so damn hip to the ways of the white man — and so Black — playing divine music to Miss Ann's naked behind?" Mimi had protested. But no one was taken with what she had to say as if she had become soundless as the epoch had faded.

A move to the East Coast and a fractious divorce led me to become Buddhist. Thereupon, I began to examine my predilection for turmoil, violent upheavals, and severing ties with people. It was sobering. Other people, society, my parents, and lovers ceased being my culprits. It took deep self-reflection to face the culprit within.

Genre: Short Stories

- The protagonist of "Making Room" is haunted by an apparition of her aborted baby. The paranormal becomes the norm as she tries but can't shake off the residue of her long-ago act.

- In "Hometown Buffet," an elder subjects her granddaughter once more to a telling of a rape and subsequent childbirth way back in 1936. She adds details that shift the granddaughter's perception of the rape.

- "Sorors," a dark take on joining a Greek organization, sees two generations divided. An overbearing mother who has achieved the milestones of Black middle-class respectability forces her pregnant daughter to do the same. But the daughter, in a shocking act of personal rebellion, would rather overturn the system than rise to its upper ranks.

- In "When Dottie Meets Ouida," Ouida and Rachman are reporters for a large newspaper in New Jersey. She has agreed to have a small dinner for his sister visiting from the South. Unbeknownst to either of them, the sister turns out to be a rabid anti-abortionist.

- "In Triplets" set in Berkeley, California, a reuniting of triplets separated during The Great Depression occurs.

"Making Room"

When I walked into my bedroom, I saw a little brown boy — cocoa brown, not much hair, big round baby head — playing in front of my son Khiron's picture. He disappeared as soon as I stepped through the door, like he was playing peek-a-boo.

It startled me. I was afraid of seeing "ghosts" of the dead, again. I hadn't seen one for a while… pretty much since I saw Dad sitting on the chair in Mom's living room, laughing his head off, his hair black and cut to the curl, like when he was on his way to the racetrack. Of course I don't count seeing Raina's mom who had died in a hospital in Gainesville on Thursday. That Friday I was skimming the freeway to be Raina's friend in her time of need, and a lady in a rickety station wagon, with doors a different color than the car, was in front of me. She looked like she'd stepped out of the kitchen in her slippers to get some milk. As she got off at my exit, she turned her head ever so slightly and I recognized her as Raina's mom. She drove off and vanished over the crest of the hill — into San Francisco Bay for all I know.

Of course I didn't mention it to Raina. You can't do that. Talk to the relative about seeing the person who just died. They'll think you're off in the head and even be insulted. Anyway, there was the time I told Raina about going out-of-body. About it being a sweltering day and lying on my bed, one minute chilling, the next, a foot above my bed, suspended, begging the spirits to let me down. Which they did after a long while, though the clock had marked only a few minutes.

Raina said, according to what she'd read, out-of-body stuff only happened at death. People don't like to think about the dead or spirits hanging around, even though they say *Jesus Christ* fifty times a day. I stub my toe. *Jesus Christ*! Uncle Sam wants another $400 from me. *Jesus Fucking Christ*. Can't you see the no left turn sign, *Jeez-us*! But I'm people too. Seeing the dead can be trying. Life is very comfortable — at least during the day — without consciously making room for the dead. I'm kind of trying not to get back to the little brown boy because he has a history, a life of his own, if you will. I will get to him because he has to be heard. The dead are persistent.

My mother taught me about the spirits when I was a girl. She said I was the only one who listened to her stories. My dad called her a Gracie Allen. Gracie was George Burns' wife and straight man. But my mother never meant to be funny. She got very hurt when people laughed at her, and she'd clam up. Whenever she was braiding or pressing my hair, though, she told the stories. Stories about growing up in Oklahoma. About Washington, DC, where she went after her graduation from Langston University and saw FDR in a parade. About first coming to California and catching the streetcars, and about being the dispatcher in Dad's cab company in Berkeley and the cabbies falling in love with her voice and wanting to take her out until they found out whose wife she was.

She told me about her Papa dying when she was the same age I was then—nine. Papa had caught tuberculosis from walking eight miles in the freezing snow to his laundry job in downtown Muskogee. The family set up his sickbed in the living room so people who had heard he was dying could pay their respects. His last night Grandmother made her go to her room. But my mom told me that in the middle of the night she woke straight up. She saw these little people, the size of children, rotund and nimble and kind of glowing, walk past her bedstead and down the hall to Papa. When they marched back through, Papa was with them. And they were walking but not on the floor — a bit above it.

Of course she doesn't tell this to every Tom, Dick, and Harry. My mom's a fifty-years-and-a-gold-watch kind of person. She was one of the first blacks to integrate the civil service — soon as FDR issued Executive Order 8802. She is Missus Solid. She pays parking tickets as soon as she gets them and never U-turns in the middle of the street.

But she knows about the dead.

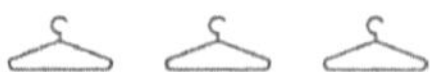

She used to get these federal credit union loans for when Dad had gambled the money into the Bay, and somehow, the way she told it, it was always a struggle. Would it be approved? Would they give her enough? Would she get to the union office before it closed? I suppose Mom was hurrying in that gray Ford with as much an eye for the loans as Dad had for his horses — Misty Light, Pretty Patty or Rump the

Roast — rounding that last lap at Golden Gate Fields. Dad kidded before he died that the only reason their marriage lasted was because they always had two cars.

On one of her trips to the credit union, she encountered someone walking down the stairs as she was going up, Mom with her worried head down, suppliant, thinking I'm sure of our five open mouths, parted like a nest of baby wrens. She said the person bumped into her, causing her to look up for a minute and see that the person was smiling. But Mom was concentrating on the loan. As soon as they passed one another, Mom realized it was a woman with "great big huge upside-down teeth." She looked back. But the woman was gone.

Of course she got the money, cashed the check, fed us, comforted us to sleep, locked my Dad out of the house for the night, and thanked the good Lord for the angel on the stairs that had been there to tell her it was all going to work out.

I still look at people's teeth like I'm going to spot divinity there. *Jesus Christ*. Like divinity is a guessing game. I hope it's not. But you do have to be on your toes to keep up with the dead. The ones I've seen move quickly. And, for some reason, I'm usually tired or stressed when they whiz by. I saw Dad streak by in a car down 69th one day, looking like Joe Louis in his prime. It reminded me of how he and Mom argued over money (do married people argue about anything else?) and he backed out of the driveway at 30 mph. Thank goodness no car was coming. When I dream of Dad, he looks like the Brown Bomber. He and Joe favored, even in old age.

Before I tell about the little brown boy, I have to tell my dad's favorite Joe Louis story.

Dad was a Tuskegee Airman, 337th, W.W.II, serving in Italy; Joe Louis back in the states was at his peak as The Brown Bomber. Dad's CO came up with a brilliant idea: get the real Joe and the look-alike Joe in an exhibition bout. Dad went along for a minute. Then, being a bright guy and knowing the real Joe wasn't famous for his smarts, my dad said to himself, what if the real Joe forgets it's a fake fight? Dad bowed out.

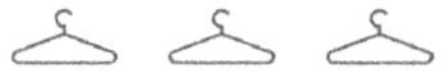

The little brown boy playing with Khiron's picture — that's what got me. I keep that picture — one of those 8 ½ by 11 school photos — next to my bedside. Khiron hates it because it's pre-braces. But I love his all-over-the-place smile; I loved that age, nine or ten, before he stopped asking, "right, Mommy?" like I knew everything,

The year before Khiron was born, I was, as we say, "out there" and had an abortion. Legal and all. But I had a hard time deciding to do it, getting a doctor, the whole bit. It was a second trimester. I guess not quite a partial birth one. But I had to go in the hospital and, in a way, deliver it. They flooded my uterus and basically drowned it, I guess. I remember asking the nurse if it was a boy or girl, and she said in a kindly tone that I didn't need to know. What can I say? I had tried to abort it myself by taking a hundred Carter's little liver pills, contemplated going to Sweden or Mexico (yeah… and my rent was $87 a month), and finally saw a shrink in Berkeley twice who then okayed the procedure. I did it, mourned it, then fell madly in love, married and had Khiron as fast as I could. I picked the name because Chiron is the god of healing. I fell in love with my baby. Adored him. Isn't that what a mother does?

"Welcome to the exquisite pain of parenting an adult," Raina tells me when I complain about Khiron — the loss of contact, the unreturned phone calls, the advice not solicited.

Exquisite pain. Yet here is the little brown boy. Ever since I moved here, I've been buying yin-yang for kids — friends' kids, anybody's kids. I have a yellow rubber ducky on the bathtub, a teddy bear and a wicker chair the height of a ruler next to the window. But my friends bring wine or cheesecake and juicy gossip. I have this picture of brown boys on the wall, playing stickball, going fishing. I cook spaghetti and bean soup — like I used to for Khiron — and throw it away, hoping rats somewhere taste my cooking and rave over it. *Jesus*, I chase enough spiders out of this place. I provide them a home — why not the little brown boy? There's even a little ceramic house on top of the bookcase for him to go in at night and rest his bones. I think the little brown boy is begging me to think of him, too. Somebody said cats spend three-quarters of their time being cats. That's why they don't pay us much mind. Maybe the dead are like that. High maintenance in their own convoluted way… *little brown boy, I'm sorry you didn't get to be loved and live a life like Khiron...* I mean, who else knows that he was playing with Khiron in the picture? Who else remembers? Who else cares?

"Hometown Buffet"

As always, Granny's face was solemn. I thought it came from answering the phone at the funeral parlor when she was young. A girl of seven or eight looking into the face of death a few hours every day. I knew someone else my age who was raised at a cemetery; her father was the groundskeeper. Her expression, soft and not quite what you'd call dour, didn't vary either. Both were caused, I figured, by similar environments.

We were sitting in Hometown Buffet in San Lorenzo, the noisiest all-you-can-eat place around. I hate it, but Granny loves the stuffing and soft chicken. And cobbler. The little kids dashing around like cars on a freeway drive me batty, but we go there twice a month. The family calls me Granny's favorite, which she shrugs off. "She's got listening ears," she'll say, mostly when she's about to talk my ear off.

After our first plate, Granny said, "I'm going to tell you something I never have told anyone."

I teased Granny about being a closet drama queen. I had to explain it, but midway through, she said, real loud, "I'm not gay," and started talking about the baby she'd had at 15. I guess I sighed—I knew all about it: the secret, the date rape, that it was a girl, that people in the next town had taken it. I got up and brought back cherry cobbler.

"I didn't tell you this. I never told anybody this." The lenses of her eyeglasses magnified the solemn look.

"Lemuel Jackson. Lem. That was the boy's name. We had met at the dance. He wasn't a Muskogee boy." Granny hadn't migrated to Oakland till the war.

"My friends Tessa and Clydie talked me into using my mother's parlor to play cards." Iona, my great grandmother, was widowed when Granny was nine. So she raised Granny and Sister by herself. She had been a teacher until the Muskogee schools upgraded. "They knew I liked him. They invited him over. We were playing whist and Lem asked me to show him the bathroom. Instead he shoved me into the bedroom and raped me. Very fast. I never saw him again."

I thought it had happened on a date, in a car. I had always pictured Granny helpless and struggling in a Model T. not at home on a bed. This seemed not as rough a plight, even though rape is rape. I asked Granny what Iona said.

"I didn't tell anyone. I was ashamed of it. I was sleeping in Iona's room and she was on the pullout couch in the front room. I just put the teddy pillow on the spot when I made up the bed.

"When did you know you were pregnant?"

"Right away I knew it. I didn't have morning sickness either. I was too scared to say something to Iona."

In 1929, Iona's husband died of TB and she had to work as a domestic in a downtown hotel. Granny kept a single picture of Iona on her dresser. She looked so strict; I know she wouldn't have approved of cards, especially for girls. Her hard smile and forbidding look reminded me of Lee Van Cleef in the spaghetti westerns. Killer tough.

"Iona was waiting for me to tell her. She knew already from Sister." Who'd gotten pregnant the year before and Granny'd witnessed the at-home abortion. I knew that story well too: the blood, the secrecy, the screams, the infection, and the doctor at the last.

"Sister came forward early enough with hers. I had seen all that blood and never wanted to go through that."

Granny asked me to get her a coffee. Walking back, I looked at how straight her back was even with the hump of age. It was after two, and the place had cleared out, leaving mostly other seniors and us. The air conditioning had been turned on. Sister — "the smart one" — had gotten a scholarship to Langston University, the black college north of Oklahoma City. I shivered at the thought of Iona staring Granny down every morning before Granny left for work.

"Clydie guessed, but she didn't say a thing, just looked at it every day at school, watching it grow. Finally I told Iona. She was calm. She put her grip down and said, 'We're going to handle this. Don't say a word to anyone. Do you understand me?' I nodded and Iona went to work, and I sat there and cried my heart out. From then on, whenever any one wasn't around, I cried."

Granny always bragged on how Iona knew everybody, black *and* white, in Muskogee, how she was a deaconess, how she had her own proverbs and the Bible's.

"Well, Iona wasn't perfect, Granny. Didn't you say she used to have a drink at night?"

Granny looked aghast. "She wasn't an alcoholic. She just kept a bottle in the closet to nip on." Her stash, her stash, I said in my head.

"Muskogee was full of black people, and while we didn't associate with white people, even the poor blacks were snooty. Now go up and get me a heel, Sweets."

I frowned. "The food's all picked over, Granny."

"Oh, don't I know it, but the children throw back the heel. That's why I love it. Nobody wants it but me."

"That's enough to turn my stomach."

"Scoot your up-turned stomach up there. And don't forget the butter."

I placed two ends of white bread and two pats of butter before her.

"Mother took me to the doctor. And after he examined me, he said to Mother, 'What makes you think she was raped?' And Mother said, 'I wasn't there. I didn't see it. But my bed was used for raping my child. How do I know? Because the bedspread had a blood spot the size of an orange.' "

Granny smiled. "Up until then I thought Mother didn't believe me."

The help, all young and mostly Latino, sat at one end of the room. Granny started nibbling on a heel.

"Mother had a friend in Sand Springs — Miss Jessie — been in a bad marriage, and when it broke up, Mother let her live with us. So Mother arranged for me to stay with Miss Jessie through the delivery. When time came — seven and a half months — Mother put me on a bus, bright and early in the morn, for Sand Springs."

Granny was getting agitated. "She gave me instructions. *The bus will go through Tulsa. Stay on it. Don't get off. Get off in Sand Springs. Go straight to Miss Jessie's. She lives a block and a half straight down*

*from the station. Stay inside Miss Jessie's and don't bother nobody.
When you have it, you're going to stay for three days. Get on your feet.
Miss Jessie will put you back on the bus. Do not bring it back with you.
Do you understand me?'* And then she repeated everything."

Granny looked around, as if some thought was coming to her. "Sweets,
go get Granny's Jell-O, please."

I went up and put three cubes in a saucer. Granny was standing when
I got back.

"Are you ready to go?"

"Stretching, child." She sat down. "You know that ride to Sand Springs
took a long while. Muskogee was a city. I was a city girl. We passed
those little towns along the Arkansas River. First Taft, where they had
the mental hospital. Then Red Bird. Colored lived there, and Bixby.
That long stretch of the Arkansas had me to thinking of Poppa. He'd
go fishing there. Drive his four-door Ford in the summer without the
windows. He kept the windows put away — all canvas, plastic and
snaps. And we'd snap them off. Every piece of window had a snap."
She sighed. It was a good memory for Granny. She told me before that
Poppa stuck up for her and that he'd been gentle.

"They had high ideals," she said. "Poor folks didn't just sit around and
be pitiful in those days. When I got to the town, I went straight to Miss
Jessie's. She had a one-bedroom house so she put me up a cot in her
room. Mostly though she was up at her white folks working. I had my
orders not to go anywhere. She'd cook, put it in the icebox, and I'd eat
off it for two or three days. I was there by myself most of the time. I'd
been told not to ask any questions and not to tell any of my business.

"Now the ice man came by every day. I'd get 25¢ worth of ice to last
two days. Miss Jessie cooked fried chicken, peas, and beans. I made
the cornbread."

I felt so bad for Granny — all alone and so naive — and I got mad at
Iona.

"There were four women who lived alongside Miss Jessie and they
were told to look in on me. The woman two doors down took a real

interest in me. Gave me ripe bananas. She wanted a baby real bad. She said to me, 'I like to have your baby. You can just give it to me when you spit it out.' I wanted to spit out the whole story, but I kept it inside.

"When my water broke, I called her and she called Miss Jessie who came right down. She had me to lie on my back and take my panties off. Then she said, 'There's nothing anybody can do right now. You're going to get these pains. Just grunt real hard to bring the baby's head down.' By time the other women came, it was out. They all washed it and by then the doctor from Sand Springs, or Tulsa I guess, got there. He cut the cord, examined it, and complimented the women. I gave him the money Mother had given me — it wasn't but about $20 — and out he went. I named her Cora Lynn. She had a beautiful high brown color and chubby cheeks, like Lem. The woman that gave me the bananas took it. July 13, 1936, I believe."

We both sighed. The room had cleared. The help had finished lunch.

"I knew what I had to do. I was to pack my things and get back to Muskogee as soon as possible. I stayed in bed for three days and then I caught the evening bus out of Sand Springs and I was glad to go. I had to finish school and get into Langston."

We walked out of the all-you-can-eat buffet. I unlocked the car for Granny.

"As slow as the ride there was, that's how fast it was going back. Those towns whizzed by. Pitch black outside. Each time I tried to think of it, I couldn't. It was like the dark covered everything, even inside my head."

Granny and I were on 880 headed back to Oakland, ahead of the commute traffic. "All these lights and neon signs. Drive the Nimitz anytime and it's still all lit up. Iona met me at the bus station. She grilled me. *'Did you do this? Did you do that.'* And I nodded where I was to nod and shook my head where to shake. Iona never mentioned it again. Sister never mentioned it at all. And I never saw Miss Jessie again."

I stayed in the slow lane like Granny preferred. I glanced at her to see if telling the story had relieved her. "How are you feeling, Granny?"

"I have a pain in my chest."

"Where in your chest?" I knew Granny was taking lopressor for her arrhythmia.

"In my heart." She touched the center of her chest.

"How long have you been feeling it?" I debated pulling over.

"Since I finished telling you. Feels like a little knife cutting a piece out for somebody to chew on."

We were halfway between Kaiser Hospital in north Oakland and the one in Hayward. "Should we go to Kaiser?"

"No, no, it's going away. I made myself forget it. It's not painful. I was underage. I had to do what I was told. I'll be okay." We passed the Oakland city line. "Hometown's chicken tastes like the chicken up in Reno."

I sped up because I was out of the suburbs. Granny told me to slow down.

"One time in that sixty years I was standing on a street corner in Oakland. A woman who would have been her age and coloring stared at me hard. So hard I thought back to Sand Springs." Granny rocked back in the seat like church, the part where the preacher gives the call. "Iona did the best she could."

When we got to Granny's senior apartment complex, she turned. Very sternly, she said, "Now that I've told you, I don't want to discuss it again."

I nodded. I walked Granny to her elevator. I went to push the button and she put her hand on mine. "I want to eat this before I go up." She pulled a napkin out of her purse and munched on a heel. When she finished, she wiped her mouth with the napkin from the buffet. She balled it up tightly. Then she balled it up again tighter, like it was clay and she was making it perfectly round.

"Since I told you everything, I might as well tell you this too, Sweets. I saw him once again. At Langston. I was with a friend and she asked me why this boy was looking at us so hard. I turned and saw it was him.

He was staring at me. I told her, 'He's not going to bother us. Don't worry.' And he turned and went in the other direction and I never saw him again."

We went up and got Granny settled in. When I said goodbye, Granny's expression looked dead on Iona's. Spitting.

Then Granny smiled, and her face went soft and solemn as always.

"Sorors"

The ten pledges stood at attention while the big sister examined their dresses with a critical white eye. Each of the ten young women wore a white wool empire-waisted jumper with a long sleeved black silk blouse, the pledge group's chosen colors.

"Your collar has a wrinkle... little sister Xavi We are not only neat, we are immaculate. We have a tradition to uphold. On this campus, we have always initiated only the best, the cream of the crop. Your individual appearance, especially during pledge week, is a statement about all of us, and all of the women who have joined this sorority. Every single soror, past, present, and future, is judged by your image."

Xavi's first instinct was to touch the collar she had carefully pressed. She smothered this instinct which would have been unquestionably impudent. She had heard that word enough this past week. It hadn't been the hardest week in her life, but in her 21 years, it had been as full of questions as any she had. Why she was pledging was the primary puzzle which she was still unable to piece together. No, why wasn't she pledging? Was this not the same sorority that thirty years ago would not allow her mother to join because she couldn't pass the paper bag test at Lincoln University, though of course she couldn't single out Lincoln as the culprit since most of the Negro colleges and schools had used the same criteria for social status: light complexion, preferably of no darker shading than a paper bag. Her mother, as dark as a roasted chestnut, had tried in vain, even waited two years for a new group of sorors to change the unspoken tradition or to make an exception in her case. After all, she did possess the exceptionally keen features and long Indian straight black hair, so highly valued by the race. But Adella, as her mother preferred to Louise which she said was a graceless name, had settled for marrying a light skinned, if uneducated man, whose genes, it was practically guaranteed, would produce a child at least half as dark as she.

Xavi had been no disappointment in that respect. An artist's skillful blending from a multihued palette could not have produced a finer yellow tone with a luster that people admired. However, Adella had been at first surprised that her baby's peach yellow face had no bridge on its nose. She set about molding Xavi's nose with her forefinger and thumb every time she looked at it. She heard people compliment her baby's beauty but saw only flatness and limitation. As black as she was, Adella had thanked the heavens everyday for keen features and straight hair. But for her baby — the one who would, dammit, be able to join any socially elite group of colored folk — to have a wide nose made her flinch. With prayer and concentration she bore the other cross, a drunken husband whose instinct during the entirety of their marriage had been to ignore her. A dentist's prosthesis rectified the gap in the front of Xavi's teeth. Ballet lessons straightened her knock knees. She was a beautiful child, after all the money, time and worry. That she was extremely bright was nice in Adella's mind, but beauty would determine all. If you had asked her to tally the net gain of her own beauty, she would have looked dumbfounded. Instead she put every whit of caring into Xavi. Xavi was salvation.

I'm paying Mama back. That's it. I'm doing this for Mama. Being a soror doesn't mean a hill of beans. Xavi had told herself this all semester. She had wanted to puke at the initiation rites. Each of them had spit into a Dixie cup. Then the soror had made them each drink from it. That had been nauseating. But a conversation she had had with one of the fraternity pledges had made her feel even weaker in the knees.

He had approached her in the commons. "I got it on the Q.T. you the next president of the white and black once you go over."

"If I get over," she retorted.

"Hey, lil' sister, ain't no doubt. Beauty, brains, fineness. If they don't let you over, the white and black would lose a lot of points with the brothers." This was the same brother she had helped through elementary chemistry. Xavi sensed that he had something to say or something to ask. He was not bright academically but he was a master at manipulation.

"All right, what else is on your mind?" She looked at him unsmilingly.

He put his hand on her head. "Your mama and your papa sho nuff gave you a pretty head of hair. Straight and black as coal."

She reached up and removed his hand. "Get to the point."

"You'd have some pretty babies, even if you married me." His laugh was hollow and mocking. Xavi tensed at the contempt in it.

"Q.T. has it," the glints in his eyes could have been crystal knives. "That the foxy president-to-be of the white and black had a baby on the strictly Q.T. and that her big sisters would be upset, why, disgraced, maybe even expelled from national if this was the absolute, verifiable truth. Can you dig it?"

An involuntary twitch. A suddenly dry throat. A soundless thud in her abdomen. Somebody knew! Somebody had found out. Adella! She wanted to pull on her mother and be protected from this sudden exposure to the cold.

"What are you talking about?" Xavi asked with a scornful air.

"Don't act dippy, everybody knows." He was trying to do her a favor; this she knew by the way his mouth was set, like he had always known. "Everybody, everybody who knows you, knows all about you. Don't you know that a secret is the only thing culled folks love to share besides food?"

Xavi gathered her books and turned away from him. He put his hand on her shoulder.

"I just wanted you to know." He walked away.

As soon as she got to her room, Xavi dialed an outside line and called Adella long distance. She related verbatim what the fraternity brother had told her.

"Now, baby, don't be too upset, that nigger might have been pulling at straws."

"But, Mama, how could he have known? Who else knew but you and me?"

There was a long pause.

"The Dean of Girls, baby."

"The Dean of Girls? How could she possibly have known?"

"Uh, I had to tell her, baby, so you couldn't have no bad mark on your record."

"Mama, I had the baby during the summer. I wasn't showing." Xavi's voice was reaching into its highest octaves. "Mama, how did the dean find out in the first place?"

"Now calm down. Remember the social worker at the home? That colored lady who was so nice to you?"

"The one who found the baby's parents?"

"Yes, dear. She thought you might need some counseling when you got back at school. Seeing as how upset you were, how you didn't want to give up the baby at first, how you was going back 'n forth between keeping the baby or giving it up. She was trying to help you, Xavi darling, that's all."

"So what did she do?"

"She wrote the Dean a letter, and sent me a copy. It was all strictly confidential."

Xavi exploded. "Strictly confidential!! To the Dean of Girls. Oh my god, no wonder everybody knows. Mama, secretaries read her mail."

"But baby, once you got back to school and started pledging, you were all right. And the Dean called and told me she tore up the letter and as far as she was concerned, she had never seen it."

"No wonder I'm the laughing stock of the whole school."

"Listen, baby, without the letter, cain't nobody prove nothing."

"Mama, that's beside the point." Her voice broke. "And to let me go through pledging knowing that everybody's got my secret on the tip of their tongues."

"Are you the first pledge with a baby off somewhere? Listen to me, Xavi, there isn't a soul on earth got a record of this. No birth certificate, no proof."

"If national finds out, it's all for nothing anyway."

"I'll take national to court on that, if need be. My baby's gonna be a soror if the walls of the Supreme Court have to shake."

"Everything is messed up, Mama."

"No, baby, everything is all right."

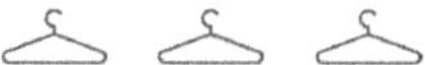

Xavi pledged, crossing the line, acting for all the world as if it was the most important thing in the world. That night, after the parties, slightly drunk, she opened the door to her dorm room. Without skipping a step, she walked over to the window and studied the grass twelve stories below. Unfastening the gold pin, the confirmation of her belonging, from her white jumper, Xavi threw it past the ledge and slammed the window shut.

Then she went into the bathroom, removed all the bobby pins from her hair and brushed her straight black hair for a long while, careful strokes from scalp to shoulder and out. When she finished, she took the scissors and cut it all off. When she was done, she looked into the mirror and stared for a while at her flat nose, her thin wide mouth and high forehead.

The next day she mailed a package, filled with the long severed strands of hair, from the campus post office to her mother.

"When Dottie Meets Ouida"

With oven mitts, Madeira carried the large red Dutch oven from Ouida's kitchen through the hall to her table. She put it on the buffet. At Ouida's, Rachman called to say that he was stuck in traffic on the Garden State Parkway. His cousin lived in Egg Harbor Township, where the sister was staying. Noni and Rodney came up the stairs into the hallway, filthy and ashy from swimming at Graydon Pool.

"Each of you, shower before company gets here," Madeira said. "And lotion up after."

"Together? Ew," Rodney said, going left. Noni turned right into her apartment.

"You know that's not what I mean," Madeira said.

She called after them." This lamb stew is smoking, kiddos."

Ouida was talking loud enough so Madeira could hear. "Which exit are you near, Rachman? Please tell me you're not just starting out. Egg Harbor Township is 134 miles away, two hours and 15 minutes. I have food on the table."

He gave her the Parkway exit. She shrieked. "That's Clifton! You're almost here. Okay, hurry, hurry. I mean don't break any laws. I'm really looking forward to meeting your sister."

Madeira took a spoon and dipped into the Dutch oven. "This is so good. Please show me how to make it. How did you get just the right amount of spiciness, Ouida?"

"African pepper paste from that store in Brooklyn." She went back to her kitchen to fix platters of basmati rice and sweet potato biscuits.

By the time she came back with platters in both arms, everyone had converged in the hallway — Rachman, his sister, Madeira welcoming them into the door of the dining room, both kids fresh from showering. Rachman was confused as to which door.

Ouida directed him. "We're doing it at Madeira's. We can sit and eat together around the table."

"Dottie's my sister from Georgia," Rachman said as they went to seats around the table. She could have passed for Pearl Bailey, high cheekbones, fine brown color, sparkling black eyes. She had a clear Southern drawl and can-do energy.

"Thank you for having us," Dottie said to Ouida as she put her purse down.

Madeira asked Noni to show Dottie to the bathroom to freshen up. Ouida took Rachman to the kitchen to wash his hands. He gave Ouida a kiss on the cheek.

Madeira said from the dining room, "Do I get one of those, too?"

He came back into the dining room, bent down to kiss her and said, "Thanks for hosting this. I'm grateful."

Madeira showed each person where to sit. She had added two leaves to her round oak table. Ouida scooped the lamb stew into Madeira's gold-rimmed china bowls. The sweet potato biscuits and the rice in platters she placed next to cilantro, lime wedges, and sliced papaya in small saucers. Cut-glass wine and water glasses set every plate, sparkling water for Noni and Rodney.

"What a beautiful table," Dottie said to Ouida.

Ouida said, "It's all Madeira's doing, I did the cooking."

Dottie turned to Madeira and repeated her compliment. Madeira nodded with pride. They all sat down. Dottie drew her hand to Rachman on her left and grabbed Noni's on her right.

"Let us pray," Dottie said. She closed her eyes and started praying. Rachman bent his head. No one else did. Rodney looked at his mother, whose eyes were open. He crossed his eyes at her as Dottie continued to pray and turned to Noni whose eyes were wide open. The two stifled giggles. When Dottie finished, she said, "And let us all say amen."

Only Rachman said it. Dottie said, "Y'all don't pray before you eat, I see."

"Mommy only does it at Grammy's," Noni said. "And we never do it here."

"That's no way to raise up chi'ren," Dottie said. "Bless the food before you eat, that's righteousness. This ain't a Christian house?"

Rodney said, "No, ma'am, it's a Buddhist house."

Dottie looked askance at Rachman. "What in God's name does that mean? And please call me Missus because I am very proud to have been my husband's helpmeet. That's Missus with a capital M."

Rodney explained what they chanted and Dottie shook her head several times. Ouida and Madeira passed the rice and lime wedges around. Noni and Rodney began to gorge on the papaya. Rachman poured wine for Ouida and Madeira.

"Dottie," he asked. "I don't know if you drink wine."

"Yes, I do. I enjoy life," she said. He poured her a glassful.

Noni and Rodney looked at her as she took a sip. When she relaxed, they looked at ease. When she took a few more sips, they began to eat their stew

"Rachman and me didn't really spend more than three years in the same household, did we, little brother?"

"Yep, from when I was eleven to fourteen. Then you moved to your mother's."

"In Georgia where I got my good Christian training. My father, Rachman's father, was not a God-fearing man, I hate to say," she said. "Nor your mother."

"He was a very good man, Dottie," Rachman said. "Hard working, great provider. We never lacked for anything. My parents were very good people, Dottie."

"But they didn't hold the tenets. On glory day, where will they be, Rachman? Man don't live by bread alone."

"Mommy, I'm so glad you made my favorite. Sweet potato biscuits," Rodney said. He buttered one generously.

Noni said, "I didn't know you're supposed to butter them. They're delicious alone."

"Noni. Butter. Scrumptiliocious," Rodney said. "You'll never eat another one without it."

"Everything is delicious, Ouida," Rachman said. "You and your mother can burn."

"I agree. This is the best lamb stew, in fact, the best stew I've ever tasted," Dottie said. "You put your foot off in this, Ouida."

"Mommy, stand up and take a bow," Rodney said, "That's what Mommy does when she cooks a really good meal. She has to stand up and I applaud."

"And what else do we do?" Ouida stood up and bowed. Everyone clapped.

"I wash the dishes," Rodney said. "Good meal means good clean up."

As Madeira cleared the plates she said, "There's a little bit more. My little surprise."

She went into her kitchen and called to Ouida, "Get those porcelain green bowls from the sideboard."

She came back with a container of sherbet.

"It's organic. Everything we ate, as much as I could make it, is organic."

The kids went nuts.

Dottie said, "Why are people so eager to eat grass-fed? Where do dogs love to piss? The grass. Love to poop? Grass."

"Big sis, cows graze all day on grass. Have you given up beef?" Rachman asked.

She harrumphed her answer.

Rachman poured more wine for Dottie, Ouida, and Madeira. He refrained from more for himself.

"I have the long drive back, ladies. No more wine but I'll have sherbet to my heart's delight," he said.

Rodney asked Ouida, "Can we take our ice cream into Noni's bedroom? We want to play Nintendo. Please."

"Go on, go on, be careful not to spill your dessert," Ouida said.

"Mommy, can I unbutton the top button on my pants and just let my stomach hang out?" Dottie mimicked Rodney's tone. "You young women are spoiling these children to death. Do they ever get the rod?"

Madeira said, "You mean, beat them?"

"Yes, that's exactly what I mean. Spare the rod, spoil the child," Dottie said.

"Do you beat your children, Dottie?" Madeira asked.

"I don't have any children. I had three miscarriages," Dottie replied. "But if I had I wouldn't spare the rod,"

"I'm sorry for your losses," Madeira said. "I'm studying nursing. I know that miscarriages are hard, especially multiple."

"I got through it with the Lord," Dottie said. "That's why it breaks my heart to see people with children raising them the wrong way."

"Whoa, Dottie," Rachman said. "That's a blanket indictment. Ever heard of live and let live."

"Not when the devil's active."

Noni and Rodney came back through with their empty dishes. Rodney announced, "We're doing the dishes now. I'll wash, and Noni's drying."

"This is foolish. They don't say grace, they eat all over the house, and they tell you when they're going to do chores? This is backwards," Dottie said.

Rodney walked past and tossed a comment to Noni. "Have they started on politics or religion yet? That's when the arguing starts."

"Young ladies," Dottie said. "I'm not here to argue, but I call it like I see it."

"Let's talk about Rachman. He just got a new job at the paper. He's a fulltime reporter. That's a big leap," Ouida said.

Rachman said, "I was letting you women go at it. Since I don't have a fellow to back me up, I'm outnumbered."

"Rachman, what's your next feature assignment?" Ouida asked, cheerily.

He hesitated, looking like a deer caught in the headlights. "Abortion."

"Abortion. I'm against abortion," Dottie said. "Why are they assigning you that?"

"It's in the news, abortion clinics are being set on fire, lives threatened," he said.

"They should be set on fire," Dottie said.

Ouida said, "Dottie, that involves potential loss of life."

Rodney came back in to clear up more dishes. "Politics or religion, right?"

"I've lost three babies. Why would I support killing babies on purpose?"

Madeira said, "Do you support abortion in cases of rape or if the mother's life is threatened?"

"No, absolutely not."

"Dottie, I wrote a column about a twelve year old girl who was raped by an older brother," Ouida said. "Her social worker had to go to court to get the judge's permission to abort because her mother wanted her to have the baby. At twelve."

"There's nothing wrong with having a baby at 12. Plenty people start out young. Even younger than that," Dottie said, her arms folded across her chest. "I'd take her baby and raise it by myself."

"You and your husband, then, do offer to adopt or raise babies from situations like that?" Ouida asked.

"My husband left me after I couldn't produce children. He didn't want a barren woman."

Ouida sighed, "Dottie, Dottie, you support right wing fanatics."

"Yes, I do, all the way. I picket those clinics in Georgia."

Rachman said, "Those anti-abortion people bomb clinics, they commit arson. It's only a matter of time before they kill someone. They've threatened to shoot doctors who perform abortions."

"Yes, I support all that. My pastor said our children are our future. When you go in and kill those fetuses, you're killing the future. It has to be stopped. And this is not up for debate," Dottie said, with finality. She turned pointedly to Ouida. "And your husband? What happened there? Rachman said you're divorcing."

Ouida got up and went out into the hall, Rachman followed her out.

Madeira answered before she got asked the same. "Dottie, I can tell you I have no desire to be married again. Marriage infantilizes women. They act only at the mercy of their husbands."

"Nonsense. Y'all young and healthy. You should be married," Dottie said. "Especially with children. Set the example."

In the kitchen Ouida spoke in a low voice. "She's crazy, Rachman. Did you know this? How could you have not known this?"

"She slept all the way up."

"Didn't she say something on the way here?"

"We haven't seen each other since we were kids," he said. Ouida threw up her hands and walked back in.

Madeira said, "And she just accused Rachman of being gay."

"What?!" Rachman said. Rodney and Noni were standing in the doorway listening to everything, dishtowels in hand.

Dottie got up and wagged her finger in Rachman's face. "You know you used to go the pond with the boys and y'all would masturbate in a circle. I heard all about it. That's homosexuality, Rachman. You're a sissy."

"Dottie! Where is all this coming from? That's called a circle jerk. Every Southern boy living in the woods does that at one time or another. It's not homosexuality. It's having fun."

"Fun! You touched each other's privates. You made each other come to climax."

"Not all the time. Sometimes we would just try to see who could shoot their shot the farthest."

"Eww. Eww. Eww," Noni said. She and Rodney went back to the dishes, laughing their butts off.

"Why are your children laughing about all this disgusting talk? You as mothers should be horrified." Dottie said, grabbing her purse. "My pastor teaches us about it, Rachman. And you used to do it all the time. You never got married, you don't have children. Isn't there some connection between other boys touching your penis and you spilling your seed on the ground?"

"Dottie, why are you grabbing your purse?" Ouida asked. "Do you feel threatened?"

"I'm ready to go."

"Let's all sit down and calm down," Ouida said. She didn't want the children to see adults fighting over ideas. Ideas, she knew, had to be aired out on some level. Talked out. Besides, it pained her to think of Rachman having to drive for two hours and 15 minutes in the car with Dottie in this state.

"Let's go back to the subject of doctors and the abortion clinics, okay?" Ouida said. Rachman poured wine into the cut glasses half-full.

"Pastor said when these young girls keep getting abortions, it destroys their hope for the future. And it affects everybody in the family. Everybody knows when they do it. I live in a small town. These girls go to Planned Parenthood but they don't stay overnight. They come home, after outpatient surgery. We used to call it D & C. They would scrape the baby out of the uterus. Now they just give them an injection and the baby comes out in blood clots. But they clot all night, the next day. Sometimes all weekend. Their parents, the sisters in the church, we have to administer to them. There's no fancy nancy way of doing it. We have to watch over them because what happens if they bleed to death? We can't let that happen. So they're making us partners to abortion, I don't like it. That's not right."

"You're making a valid point about aftercare," Madeira said. Rodney and Noni were listening to every word. They had stopped washing or drying and were standing breathlessly without budging in the kitchen.

"I did interview a young woman who had seven abortions, and she said she had a friend who had fifteen abortions, all through Planned Parenthood," Ouida said. "I find that alarming. It means they're using abortion as a method of birth control."

She turned her head to Rachman. "Pete killed that column idea."

Rachman smirked. "Family newspaper."

"Have either of you had an abortion?" Dottie asked Ouida and Madeira. Madeira shook her head.

"I haven't," Ouida answered. "But I believe in the right to use that option. I know about the pain and suffering that back alley abortions caused. Abortion is in the Bible, right along, right next to infanticide, Dottie."

"Where? You have to tell me where." Dottie demanded, still clutching her purse.

"Pharaoh and King Herod ordered the mass abortion of male children. That's in Exodus 1. Under Pharaoh 's command, sex-selective infanticide and abortion were used to control the Hebrew population. Midwives were instructed to abort all newborn males 'on the birthstool.' That's Exodus 1:16. In Matthew 2, King Herod hears that the 'King of the Jews' was born. Herod demanded the life of every male child two-years-old and under. That's Matthew 2:16-18."

"How can you know all this?" Dottie asked.

"She has a photographic memory, Dottie," Rachman said.

"What is that?" Dottie said. She put her purse down and sat on the sofa near the table.

"The capacity to recall information or visual images in great detail," Rachman said. "That's what makes her a great reporter."

"Please explain sex-selective infanticide," Rodney said from the kitchen.

"I got that," Rachman said. "It's also called son preference. In some cultures, children take care of the elders. However, while daughters marry and join their husband's family, the sons are supposed to support the aging parents because they have more resources. That kind of culture takes female babies and starves them to death, and other horrible things to get rid of them."

"I'm supposed to take care of you when you get older, Mommy?" Rodney asked. "Uncle Claude isn't taking care of Grandma."

"That's in some cultures, India, for example." Ouida answered. "My father left Grandma with a pension to take care of her old age."

"Will you explain back alley abortion?" Noni said, standing at the door. "That sounds like the woman squats in an alley and has a baby like an animal at the zoo or something."

Madeira said, "I'll handle that one. Before abortion was legalized by the highest court in the land in 1973, women who wanted to abort went to doctors who did the operation in unsanitary rooms. They paid a lot in cash, and sometimes the doctors didn't do it right. Like Dottie said, sometimes, the women would bleed to death because it wasn't sterile."

Dottie covered her eyes, "I bled for days after my miscarriages. That's why he left. He got tired of the smell of blood on me."

"Dottie, you went through deep trauma," Ouida said. "That has a lasting impact. Put your legs up, Dottie, Get comfortable."

"No man would want me. I'm defiled. I'm not even 40 and my life as a woman is over," Dottie said.

"Dottie, if you shoot a doctor, then your life will be over," Ouida said. "Many women face life without a mate or the ability to have natural children. They go on. They lead full lives. They work. They contribute to society in positive ways. They adopt. Or they become mothers in a broader sense, in their communities. There are always alternatives."

"But if you shut down, you can't see the good alternatives," Madeira said. "Blowing up a clinic is a bad alternative. What if one of your church members was doing janitor duties when the clinic got set on fire? And he couldn't get out in time?"

"Madeira, she fell asleep. Dottie fell asleep," Rachman said. Madeira spread a quilt over her.

Rachman and Ouida went into the hall.

"My god, she's rabid. Do you think we had any impact on her?" Ouida said.

"I don't know. She listened, especially when you quoted scripture, chapter and verse. That was genius, girl," he said.

"What can I say? Sometimes the brain power comes in handy."

"It's also seductive, you know. I like brainy women."

"Not the time or the place, Rachman."

Rodney came out into the hallway.

"Are you two getting smoochy?" he asked.

"Not today, little brother. But I like your mother," Rachman said.

"I know. But does she like you? That's always the question. Does the girl like the boy?" Rodney said.

Rachman sighed and turned to Ouida. "Thank you for your hospitality, all of it. Everyone went above and beyond. Let me wake up sis and get on the road."

"Triplets"

I'm just ahead of the police going down Telegraph in two long parallel lines to the campus. They're going to a demonstration at Cal. I'm going to Lila's Lilac Garden at the border of Oakland and Berkeley. I like Lila with her lilac dusters that she insists we wear when we're working. On 63rd St., the Alameda County sheriffs bear down so hard on their motorcycles they look like beetles, black on black on silver and black. I look up toward the Campanile on campus, down towards downtown Oakland; each way, the sidewalk's crowded. The last time I saw this was President Kennedy's motorcade.

I pass in and out of clots of bodies, squeezed between some white kids in cut off jeans, a woman in a tie-dye dress with a Lhasa Apso, the shopkeepers, more people walking dogs, and sundry black people. Black Berkeleyites. Small shop owners. Grew up in Oklahoma or Texas. Came here during WWII. Worked in the shipyards. Lived in rooming houses. Stayed on, saving pocket change in Mason jars. Opened businesses. Nothing big. Restaurant. Shoe repair shop. Two-cab taxi biz. Five and dime. Fresh fruit stand. Bought bungalows in Berkeley or East Oakland. Raised kids. Still getting up saying good morning like Lila.

Lila owns, runs, and counts the day's receipts. "Long ago and far away," she loves to say, or "women are big and men are small" or "Okies are education and Texas is family." I like her hairy legs. She will not shave her legs for anything. I like that she's taller than I am, a full inch. I look for Lila in the clots. Instead I see The Girls in dusters. The Girls are not really hers; they're only ten years younger than she is. She took them in when the institution shut down. She calls them The Girls, always "C'mon, Girls" or "Now, Girls." The Girls wave me down. The police have passed now. They were closer than bark on a tree. The Girls are making over a newspaper.

"Why are you chattering like magpies?" I ask.

"Miss Lila found our picture in the newspaper. We're in the news." They talk like a pair of radios tuned to slightly different frequencies. Annette and Arletta.

"I'm afraid to ask why."

"We're not in trouble, Geniece." They call me GEE-niece instead of juh-NIECE. "The newspaper says we're going to meet our sister."

Lila comes out and motions them back into the shop.

"Did you see the police, Lila?" I ask her.

"Seen police all my life," Lila says. "Nothing new under the sun."

"They're going to arrest the demonstrators. That's new."

"Police and demonstrators. Please. These motorcycles don't compare to a battalion of horses riding your front yard. Stomping down a good crop of mustards." She clips dead leaves from the potted plants.

Arletta shoves the paper between Lila and me. *The Berkeley Post*, the black weekly, has their picture on the first page. I read the story out loud. How Lila took them in, noting that the birth of multiple children in the Depression was a catastrophe. The Girls were farmed out, two of them to one family, the third to another.

The Girls squeal and hop around the little shop. For as long as I've known them, it was rumored they were triplets. It seems the parents who took the third one have died now and authorities undertook a search for the next of kin. They found Annette and Arletta through a mental retardation registry. The third girl was coming to Oakland.

"We have a sister. We knew it. We have a sister. The paper says our sister is coming to see us."

The picture is grainy. Her name is Trissie. The Girls go on and on. Lila takes the paper and puts it under her arms, clipping stems for the church bouquets all the while.

"Now Girls, let's wait for the moment to get excited." They pay her no mind. She keeps arranging bromeliads for display. She turns to Arletta. "Go get me some of the small pine bark."

Lila and Arletta make over the bromeliads, a specialty plant. Lila says she likes bromeliads because most people consider them strange and hard to grow.

"For the tillandsia, or the cryptanthus, Miss Lila?" Arletta turns to me on her way from the soil keeper. "Geniece, we're trying to make more of the puppy bromeliads. When they sprout, you can take one home as soon as the mother plant dies. O.K.?" I nod.

"But not before it dies."

"I heard you, Arletta."

"It leaves so many pups behind. But the mother dies."

"I know, Arletta."

"Miss Lila says I put my heart and soul in my bromeliads. Didn't you, Miss Lila?" Lila nods and starts in with the grapes. She puts a bunch in the freezer for an hour and rolls them in powdered sugar. She pops them right in our mouths because our hands are usually deep in dirt.

"That's right," Lila says. "Arletta puts Arletta's heart and soul into bromeliads." Childlike, Annette starts repeating our conversation: *Arletta's heart and soul heart and soul bromeliads bromeliads so many pups so many pups the mother dies mother dies bromeliads bromeliads.*

I start sweeping the floor. Lila isn't paying me to stand around with my mouth wide open and yapping. The next day I try to explain having a boyfriend to the Girls.

"Do you satisfy him?"

"I want to discuss things with him, Arletta."

"And all he wants is one thing, Geniece?" Annette says.

I shrug as if to say, who knows. I don't know if either of The Girls has had sex. I don't think so. They look like they're my age, not in their forties. Lila told me that's because of their condition. Their word for sex is *satisfied.*

"Maybe if you give him the one thing, he will discuss the other thing. He needs *satisfied.*"

"I think he would want *satisfied* over and over," Arletta says. "And over and over." They start repeating. *Satisfied.* And *over and over.*

"Girls?" They stop. "Do you know what a virgin is?"

They nod.

"I'm a virgin. And I don't want to be one any more."

"Like when you cut your hair off," Arletta says. Their eyes had widened when they saw me with a natural for the first time. Lila sends them for weekly press and curl.

"Yeah, like that." For a few days, they touched my hair as if it was fire.

They get into a nodding contest, repeating *virgin, don't want to be one anymore, virgin, don't want to be one anymore*. They don't look stupid to me. This is what they do — repeat any new word or concept, keep their pocket change in handkerchiefs. When they repeat these words, it has a different effect on me. Being a virgin has been my choice. I want to see what it's like not to have that choice. We finish the day's bouquets.

Annette says, "Go home and take a bath, Geniece. You stink."

The next week a reporter from the Oakland Tribune comes to the shop with a younger photographer. "How exactly did the two of you come here from Oklahoma in the first place?" the reporter asks The Girls. He's white, balding, with freckles covering his forearms, face and scalp. The photographer is mute as if his camera is mouth enough.

"We came here on a train, the Santa Fe," Arletta speaks up. The reporter smiles and fiddles with his pencil.

"No, I mean the circumstances," he says. I want to jump in and tell him how they got here, but I don't know. I want Lila to talk, but she is indifferent to their presence. When she told me they were coming for the story, she said she didn't care what the Oakland Tribune wrote. *"We made the Post, that's what counts, that damn Tribune insults my intelligence whenever it runs a story making Negroes look like buffoons."*

"We came to Oakland because our family was here," Arletta says. They didn't have family here; I knew that much. "Our poppa came here first and sent for us."

"When was that?" the reporter writes it down.

Arletta looks at me. "When we got older."

Irritated as hell, he looks at her and then the photographer. "Jesus, this is a joke." He puts his steno pad away and walks out of the shop. "Let's get the hell out of here."

When the two get into a dusty orange Ford Fairlane up the street, Lila comes out. We stand there watching them make a U-turn and head towards downtown Oakland. Arletta and I wave, but only the photographer nods. The Girls and I giggle.

"Humph, " Lila says. "Peckerwoods."

I turn to her. "Where *did* they come from, Lila?"

"Their people in Okmulgee took care of them as long as they could. When I heard The Girls needed a home, they were on the next train. You can't be colored and alone."

The second Tribune story never appears. But the third Girl comes in like rain. At first a few sprinkles, then a deluge. Lila is wired that she's on the way and we all go to the Southern Pacific Depot to pick her up. We pile in Lila's Buick Skylark. Its seats are so high and filled with horsehair we float above the streets of West Oakland. Once we pass Market Street, I can feel, just barely, the railroad tracks. Annette and Arletta play on the street names. *Myrtle, the old maid. Filbert, big fat nut. Look at that Chestnut Street roasting on the open fire. Sweet Adeline.* We pass DeFremery Park with the huge Victorian house in the center. *Here come more trees. Poplar. Cypress.* Lila points out Esther's Orbit Room and Breakfast Club like we have all the time in the world, which we do since Lila is exceedingly punctual.

"Some of these places — you'd never understand what a big deal it was." Lila's voice sounds teary, like when people sing *Lift Every Voice and Sing.* "Earl Fatha Hines whipped a mean organ in Esther's."

"When you used to be young, Miss Lila?" Annette asks.

"Young my eye. When life was a grand adventure."

Lila turns onto Campbell and finds a park across the street from a hulking, granite building. Three giant arched windows across the front look like glass portals to the San Francisco skyline.

"This is it, Girls."

I don't know whether Lila is talking about the building or coming to get Trissie.

We walk single-file like ducks behind Lila into the waiting room, past six feet tall cast iron lampposts marked Geo. Cotter Co., South Bend, Ind. And on past sculptured fountains, stone fruits and leaves cascading down pilasters, and lintels topped with large gilt crests. There aren't any people, only oak benches and marble under our feet. The heels of our shoes make clicking sounds across the floor.

Annette walks to a pedestal. "How come this looks like the cemetery?"

"Look, Miss Lila! Acanthus leaves way up," Arletta points to the ceiling three stories high.

"Arletta, how can you see that design from way down here?" I ask.

"Oh, my, Arletta is right. They call it Beaux Arts, Girls. It's used in many public places," Lila says, looking up.

"Like City Hall?" I ask.

"Like City Hall, Miss Geniece." Lila is not acting at all like herself today, calling me miss and getting teary about old, dilapidated West Oakland.

"We used to come in here all decked out for our beaux going off on the hog head run. The night run. We would go to the old waterfront terminal, and board the ferry to Frisco. They had an orchestra on the ferry," Lila starts humming. Annette starts saying, *Bo, Bo, little Bo peep lost her sheep, lost her sheep.*

"Can you imagine?" Lila talks over Annette. "On a ferry on the San Francisco Bay listening to a white band playing Count Basie. Oh! This California. We left the South in the dust. And after we got back on this side of the bay, our fellas would put on their porters' uniforms and we'd take their dress clothes home. Now that was grand."

The train whistles somewhere far as if it had a baritone in its steel throat.

The Girls say, "Geniece, let's go up there."

We walk out to the platform, but I stand back. The Girls stand alarmingly close to the track. Why doesn't Lila pull them back? Does she want them to fall in front of the train and be crushed to death? Lila stands next to me, holding her car keys like prayer beads, looking for the locomotive and sighing. I feel the train's rumble in the concrete beneath me like a quake. I whisper to Lila, "is this going to drive you nuts, three of them?" I think about it, about how strong she is and how she's managed the shop and The Girls so many years. As the train whistles in, she says, "Sometimes you choose your cross, sometimes it chooses you."

A stream of passengers unlike the one we're looking for pours out. It is not hard to spot Trissie. She steps out, squinting at the sun. She puts one gloved hand up to her brow and holds her bag in the other. The Girls go up to her, Arletta leading. I can't hear what Arletta is saying because her back is to me. I make a move toward them, but Lila puts a hand on my shoulder. She doesn't speak, but her body warmth says, *let them be*. I let them, even though curiosity is killing me. I wanted to see the look on The Girls' faces when they first met her. They stand there as if time has taken a five-minute break. Then another five minutes. I can't tell who's talking. Their heads are bobbing like doll heads. I want to turn their heads around like doll heads and have them talk to me.

Finally the three of them turn and walk towards us, Trissie in the middle. Trissie has the same exact leaf brown skin, and wide set, saucer brown eyes, same size and build. But she has on black patent heels and they're wearing flats. They're in cotton seersucker pants and white blouses. Her dress is gabardine. A wide black patent leather belt emphasizes her waist. They look so much alike and unalike, it's altogether a shock.

She greets us, extending a gloved hand. "Miss Lila, I am so pleased to meet you." Good googa mooga, she has a Texas accent a mile wide. We walk to Lila's car. The Girls keep Trissie between them, as if she's a balloon that could fly away right in the back seat of the Skylark. I turn around as the car hits the streets of West Oakland.

Annette says, "The street names are trees, Trissie. Poplar. Cypress. Oak."

She turns to Trissie, "Why do you talk so funny, Trissie? Like Gomer Pyle?"

Arletta reaches across Trissie and pops Annette on the forearm. "She's southern. Don't make fun. I like it."

"Linden. Wood. Look, there's the 62 bus," Annette points to the bus. Trissie turns her head and looks back like it's no big thing.

"Trissie," I say, "your outfit looks fine after all that traveling."

"That's what they taught us at college. How to keep the press no matter how hot it gets. I starched and folded everything in my suitcases."

She sits back and relaxes into the seat. Her dress rides up and we can see she has on a white panty girdle. Her stockings are lighter than her skin. Annette runs her hand over the top of Trissie's knees. "Geniece dips our stockings in coffee so they match our skin."

Lila begins her interrogation. "You went to college, Trissie?"

"Yes, ma'am."

"Oh, such manners. Where, dear?"

"Lane College. It's my alma mater."

"What a treat, Trissie. Lane's choir is singing at our church."

Trissie sits up straight on the hump. "Down south — colored folks — we suck up education."

Suck up education, Annette repeats, suck up education.

"You went to college?" Arletta asks.

Annette repeats *suck up education, suck it up.*

"Don't look at Trissie like she has trumpets in her ears, Geniece." Arletta rolls her eyes at me.

"I'm not looking at her like anything," I turn around facing front.

Arletta asks, "Was it hard?" I turn back around. Trissie takes off her gloves finger by finger. Her nails are trimmed and polished with clear pink shellac. Primly she says, "Perseverance is the soul of success."

"Geniece said soul is a feeling," Annette says and starts singing "Soul Man" by Sam and Dave.

"I kept my nose to the grindstone."

Annette takes the ungloved hand and places it on her leg. "Look. We have the same hands."

We look at the hands while the car crosses San Pablo Avenue. It's true. All their hands are long and the joints spindly. Arletta's nails are nibbled to the quick. Annette's are short and lined at the bed with dirt from potting plants.

"A woman's nails should be neat and above all clean," Trissie says. She gives Annette a pat on the last word.

Lila says, as she turns onto Telegraph, "To each his own, my dear."

"Are you retarded like us? " Annette asks Trissie.

Arletta says quickly, "We're not retarded. I told you, we're slow."

"In the South," Trissie says, "colored are always getting labeled and then thrown in a garbage can. But I'm not retarded. Nobody threw my brain away. I bet you're not retarded either, Annette."

"Yes, I am."

"No, we're not," Arletta says.

"I like being retarded. I don't have to do as much," Annette says.

Arletta picks up Trissie's glove and runs her fingers over it. "No we're not."

"Yes, we are and I don't care." Annette begins to repeat, *nobody threw my brain away.*

"Do you want to try it on?" Trissie asks Arletta.

"I want to try them both on." Arletta pulls the glove over the palm of her hand and flexes her gloved fingers. She holds one up for us to look at, and then pulls on the other. She holds up her hands, flutters them, and folds them primly.

"Nobody in this car is retarded, okay, Annette?" Arletta says. "Not a soul."

"Geniece said soul is a feeling," Annette begins to repeat *soul is a feeling, nobody is retarded, not in this car, not a soul.* Arletta gives the gloves back to Trissie.

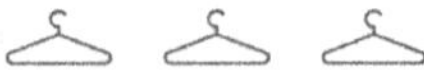

I'm late for Lila's church program, too late to meet them at the flower shop. I go directly to Lila's church, which is decked out as grandly as if it's Christmas. They've hung streamers with the names of the three black colleges — Lane, Houston-Tillotson and Wiley — which have sent singers for a joint chorale program. Sitting in my aisle seat I feel the waves of music, altos, sopranos, baritones, and the crescendo of the pianist mixing gospel with the classical strains of James Weldon Johnson. *In dat great gittin' up morning* makes me so happy I talk to myself like The Girls. Nonsensical phrases *I matter, we matter, I mattered, I mattering* echo in my head, mingling with the chorale pieces.

At intermission, I go with Trissie to her alma mater table. Trissie goes to the bathroom. I sign my name on the Lane College recruiter's list.

"Are you in high school or college already?" The woman behind the table asks. I proudly tell her college. She frowns slightly and I begin to tell her about my major and my grades.

"You don't pay tuition at a junior college?"

When I tell her I pay $2 a semester, she raises her eyebrow. "Are your parents alumna?"

My mouth drops open. I don't know what to say. I don't pay tuition. My grandmother raised me. I can't come up with the right answer. Some other students come up to the table and finger the brochures. She begins speaking to them, her voice lighter. I don't want to think about why she's nicer to them. *I matter.* I look down at the program.

Trissie walks up and says with a flourish to the woman, "All is not lost that is not forgotten hence." Then she extends her hand to the woman. The woman makes a slight bow with her head and rises to embrace Trissie.

"Young lady, what good things has been your lot since you left us?" the woman says. I want to correct her and say *have* not *has*.

Trissie says, "I've been working in floral design and sales, both here and in Oklahoma." I don't know if Trissie is blowing smoke out of her ears or what. She hasn't been here a week. We don't design at Lila's; we dig up dirt and mealy bugs and spray dieffenbachia and bake the dirt to kill the bacteria.

"Are you using your degree, child?" the woman asks her. "That's the important thing. Use your education to better yourself."

"I am. I assure you, I am," Trissie answers confidently.

The woman points to a stack of yearbooks. "What year did you graduate, dear?"

Trissie looks uncomfortable. She pulls her hands together and fingers the spines of the yearbooks. "My year isn't in here, I don't believe."

"Nonsense," the woman says. "We have every one from the last twenty years."

Trissie stammers, "I, uh, I... "

The woman stops everything — questions, shuffling of yearbooks, moving her god-awful brochures like a three-card monte. A silence grips the air.

"My dear, you aren't by chance a poseur?" she asks in a damning tone.

"What's that?"

"Someone claiming to be a thing they are not."

"I can't remember which year I –"

The woman cuts her off. "Nobody forgets the year they graduated. It's a matter of pride." She restacks the yearbooks and moves the brochures away from us. I want Trissie to leave the table, get away from this woman. I want to speak in loud, confident, clear tones. *I matter, she matters, you matter, we all matter.* Instead Trissie and I walk back to our seats, Trissie not speaking but holding her head so high.

The Girls ask, "Trissie, did you see your college table?"

That's the only time Trissie looks at me. If looks could kill, I would be in a coffin. "Uh huh.The Girls ask, "Geniece, are you going to Trissie's college?" I shrug my shoulders and we listen to "I got a home in that rock," Lila's favorite spiritual. Trissie refuses to look at me or even let our arms touch on the padded rail between our seats. Voices fill every space from the floor beneath our feet to the frescoes on the ceiling. Trissie hums the last stanza with them. As the choir members link hands for the final number, *Peace in the Valley*, the director motions the audience to link hands. Trissie and The Girls link hands. Trissie leaves her other hand at her side. I place my hand on it. Her skin is hot. She draws away from me. Her skin is unlike our hands that touch water and dirt often. I try again to take her hand. Trissie pulls her hand to her chest. I wait until she puts it down again and I grab it. But she won't close her fingers around mine. It doesn't matter. I clasp her stiff hand tightly with every ounce of feeling that I have. I can feel her hurt as if I had swallowed it. I want her to hear my heart saying *I matter, you matter*, we matter. The song ends and everyone gives the choirs a standing ovation. I turn to Trissie who looks at me for a second. When I see the pure hate in her eyes I feel a sharp pain.

⌒ ⌒ ⌒

When I come to work a few days later Lila has put Trissie on the register, something she seldom lets the Girls do.

Arletta says, with a taunting smile, "Geniece, there's nothing for you to do."

Annette says, "Go home and take a bath, Geniece, you stink."

"Do what?" It's our game. One of The Girls will say, "Do which?" But nobody answers. I look for Lila. I can hear her humming in the back.

"Trissie, can you handle it?"

"I'm good with figures. I can do it, Geniece."

Annette says, "You have to go, Geniece. Three's company, four's a crowd." Annette repeats it over and over until I correct her. Two's company, three's a crowd.

Lila's angular body fills the shop. "Is Annette right, Lila?"

"It's up to you, sweetheart," she says. She has on gardening gloves. She's been repotting. I can see there are too many bodies in here.

"Do you want to stay here, Geniece?" Lila asks.

I want Lila to say *stay here* as a command, not a question. She only asks me once. It takes a minute to feel how tiny the shop has become.

"I guess it's time for me to go."

 Lila nods and I turn to leave. Annette starts clapping.

"Annette, I thought you were my friend."

"I don't want a friend. I have my sisters and Miss Lila."

Arletta gives me a hug, Annette keeps on clapping. Trissie, popping grapes into her mouth from a brown paper bag, doesn't look me in the face. I don't want to start crying. I don't want to, but I can't help it. The tears will spill out if I blink. It's important to get out quickly.

I look at the shop from outside. The Girls and Trissie are in motion as if I had never been there. A stinging pain in the back of my throat is worse than severe thirst. It begins there and spreads. It's funny — I hate dirt and hated getting it on my hands. Lila looks up at me, shrugs and waves me on — twice, as if to say *go, find your cross, this is mine*. It eases the aching. As I turn to walk to the bus, Arletta comes out, squat-legged, carrying a terra cotta pot of the young bromeliads.

"Here, Geniece, I can grow more pups. They take less than a month." She gives me the pot, a kiss on the cheek and a Lila-style wave, and goes back in the shop.

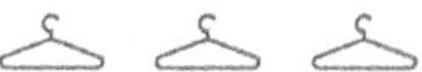

On the bus, a few weeks later, I scan the Oakland Post, the society chatter, church stories and wedding announcements. A picture looks familiar. Of all things, it's Lila's shop, a picture of the Girls and Trissie standing outside the flower shop. The triplets have on dresses cinched at the waist. They look regular, sexy, like the object of men's whistles.

As I start on the first paragraph, I can hear Lila read to all three of them in her deadpan voice. I start reading the story.

"After the reunion with her sister for the first time in 42 years, Arletta Kindler, 43, had a heart attack. By the time medics reached the scene, she had expired."

Expired. I'm thinking she fainted or stopped breathing for a minute or something. I let out a howl. People look at me like I might hurt them.

"Arletta died? How could that be?" I poke the newspaper as if it can answer me. "Damn! I read the Oakland Tribune every day. I can't believe this happened two weeks ago. Why didn't those freckle-faced, long-eared peckers have Arletta's death in it?"

Expired. I read what a Dr. Tagliablue said: "She might have been overwhelmed by the reunion with the long lost triplet. We don't know."

I catch a transfer bus to Berkeley, crying and cursing. Crying because Arletta died and cursing under my breath because I didn't know about it. Crying because I know about it and cursing because she had to die. *Damn. 43 years old.* I take the 51 bus down Telegraph Avenue, get off at 63rd St. and walk over to the shop. I stop cold in my tracks. Shouldn't I have brought something? Flowers to a flower shop? A card of condolence? I keep going. Sometimes it's enough to show your face, Lila once said over an elaborate bouquet somebody ordered. The shop's neon sign is blinking. Lila needs to fix it. I notice the green-and-white awning has a slat missing. Lila is so busy inside she probably hasn't noticed it. I pick up a discarded gum wrapper. There's no receptacle in sight. I stand directly in front of the tinted gold window. I see The Girls and Lila. The door is ajar. I hear them talking and laughing. The dusters look like lavender lab coats. Maybe I was imagining I read about Arletta. I look harder. Lila is showing them the stems of a chrysanthemum plant. She turns and sees my face. In a startled voice she says, "Oh, Geniece. No. Don't come in."

The Girls turn and see me as I come in the door. Annette starts screaming and yelling at me. Trissie tries to calm her. Their faces — Annette's and Trissie's — are too wide and open to hide the sadness. I know for sure that Arletta is dead. I keep walking into the store but Lila motions for me to back out. I back up and Annette yells out to me in guttural sobs that sound like *teef, teef.*

"She's calling to me, Lila."

"Geniece, I'm sorry, you have to go."

"I'm sorry I didn't come sooner."

"That's not the problem, sweetie."

"I would've come before now." I hear Annette saying *thief, thief.* "What's the matter?"

Lila sighs, standing on the sidewalk, and runs her fingers through the missing slot as if some portable piece of daylight had floated by.

"Sweetheart, the Girls are accusing you of stealing."

"Lila, I would never steal from you."

"Not me," she said. "Annette says you stole something from her."

I look back at Annette. Trissie is comforting her. "I need to clear this up right away, Lila." She blocks me from going in. "Lila, I'm trying to think of what Annette could possibly think I stole. Is something missing from the handkerchiefs? I'll talk to her."

"No, she gets hysterical if she thinks of you. Please, Geniece."

"But what is it she thinks I stole from her?"

"Geniece, it's not important. Don't aggravate a situation like this."

"Is it because of Arletta's death?"

Death is the wrong word. Lila looks like I hit her. I put my arm around her. She feels bony and delicate, not like the solid Lila I knew. For the first time I understand why people use words like passed away, departed, expired. I take her in both arms; her heart heaving against my chest feels like a bell swinging inside her. I sing to her, *I got a home in that rock, don't you see? I got a home in that rock.* I fight my tears.

Annette comes flying out of the shop, Trissie behind her. Annette tries to pull Lila away from me. "No, no, no, don't take Miss Lila from me."

"I'm not going to take Miss Lila from you, Annette."

"Don't steal her too, Geniece." She sobs loud enough to stop cars in traffic. "Thief, you're a thief."

"Annette, what's the matter? I didn't steal from you."

"Yes, you did. You stole Arletta. You took her bromeliads and she couldn't live without them. You stole her soul. You stole Arletta's soul." She wrenches Lila away and begins her repetitions.

"Nobody can steal your soul, Annette. It's a part of you."

Lila grips my shoulder, then lets it go and goes back in the store. *Thief, thief, you stole my sister's soul, her soul, her soul,* Annette begins screeching all the words she's learned: *nobody threw my brain away heart and soul bromeliads bromeliads you stole her soul virgin virgin coffee grind stockings suck up education suck it up satisfied satisfied satisfied.* The words sound horrible, degrading, vulgar. I look at the store, but between the sun and my blurred tears I can't see a thing. I'm being banished. The tears spill out, watering the concrete. Annette's voice follows me as I cross Telegraph Avenue to catch the bus. From the curb, she blasts all of her anguish, fury and grief at me with a set of heart-piercing shrieks:

you stole Arletta's soul you stole Arletta's soul

Genre: Poems

"the powerful nurse, the powerful baby"

da baby talks in the hospital drainage
    I coulda been a contender
    a half-baby quarter-baby
    eighth-baby sixteenth-baby
da baby sticks around
waiting for the nurse to come back
he remembers her orange dansko clogs

she can talk to the world
about how he drowned
da baby waits for her to come back
but she works four days on three days off
he's jealous of whole babies
who scream in expectation
on the other floor
he wants to join their club
    nobody wants you not even gawdzilla
da baby has to join his kind
in the sewage pipes of los angeles nyc chicago
in the pipes 22 inches below the top ground
da baby would settle to be an atonement baby
a post-war or an after three miscarriages baby
da baby wanted wholeness
he wouldn't have minded being
ugly as gawdzilla
to be alive
to eat mush and grow teeth to gather fuzz between his toes
instead of guts swirling around him

when the shift changes
da baby becomes a rush of dirty water
the drainage clears the dream of being
once and again

"It's ok Mommy"

It's ok Mommy.
I see your heart and I know just who you are.
No need to apologize, I can see your scars.
I know it was painful, but I want you to smile.
Stop your self-hate; you are innocent in my eyes.
I know my blood was a sacrifice, but you're not to blame.
Poverty is just not enough for a baby to gain.

It's ok Mommy.
Block the hatred of the world.
Replace your tears with fire.
Take the regrets out of your mind.
Because mine is full of nothing but kindness.

It's ok Mommy
Forgiveness is what I bring,
Because according to God forgiveness is life.
No need to be depressed, just live.

It's ok Mommy
I don't feel betrayed
Yes, I could have been the president,

But I could have also been a lazy river.

I could have been a doctor,

But I could have been a robber.

It's ok Mommy

Don't stay in the darkness, the light is better.

Especially when I forgive you for your tough decision.

I know there is a lot of chatter,

But I'm not in any way bitter.

Continue life and be a go-getter,

So, the next future could be brighter.

     – Jahdeen Brown

"I love hospitals. Loved them since I was a girl"

They're so clean and lit up and scary

I love hospitals. Can't stand hospital shows

This is why I love hospitals

the element of surprise

Are you gonna get better?

Are you gonna die? What?

You never know

I was one of the first people in California to get a legal abortion

umpty umpty years ago I think before roe v. wade

I don't remember. Ask my uterus still mad at me for going through menopause & getting a hysterectomy)

and I didn't even know how they were going to do it

I'm in the hospital. On my back.

alice in abortionland

What's gonna happen next?

I know how illegal abortions happen… with the doggone coat hanger
up your vagina and a ton of blood and maybe you die

I don't know how hospitals do it.

I am in a room. On my back

In a gown. Open in the front

the nurse says in a very soothing voice

    now we're just going give you a little sedative effect

      and the tissue will leave your uterus

umm, just a clot passing on

and when she says, a clot passing on, I get it

They're drowning it.

I wanted them to kill it. Not drown it

I came in for a killing not a drowning

But that's a hospital

so bright and full of surprises

so full of life and cadavers

I love em

"The philosopher"

Only two kinds of people

In this world -

daddy would grumble

as we walked
from the bus stop
and I pretended
my ankles were tied
forcing me to stumble
from lawn to lawn
—the caught and the uncaught

When my pretty catholic cousins
became pregnant
at fifteen
he handcuffed
the tiny yellow
babies into the family
I walked them
in endless circles
while the parents
went bowling
or to work

When my sister took her turn
at sixteen
he nearly bellowed
the baby out of her
promising to kill the boy.
Rocking on her belly
scabbed by turpentine
she pleaded: don't hurt
him, it was half and half

When doctors needled fluid in
to catch my mistake
he would not hear
talk of first
and second
trimesters
psychiatrists
evaluating
my state of mind.
He looked at
the gray gown
the male orderly
my dangling leg
as if he was helplessly ill
Later he said
he only wanted me to have
healthy babies
one day

Abortion he never talked about.

APPENDIX I

Genre:
Creative Nonfiction,
An Abortion
Compendium

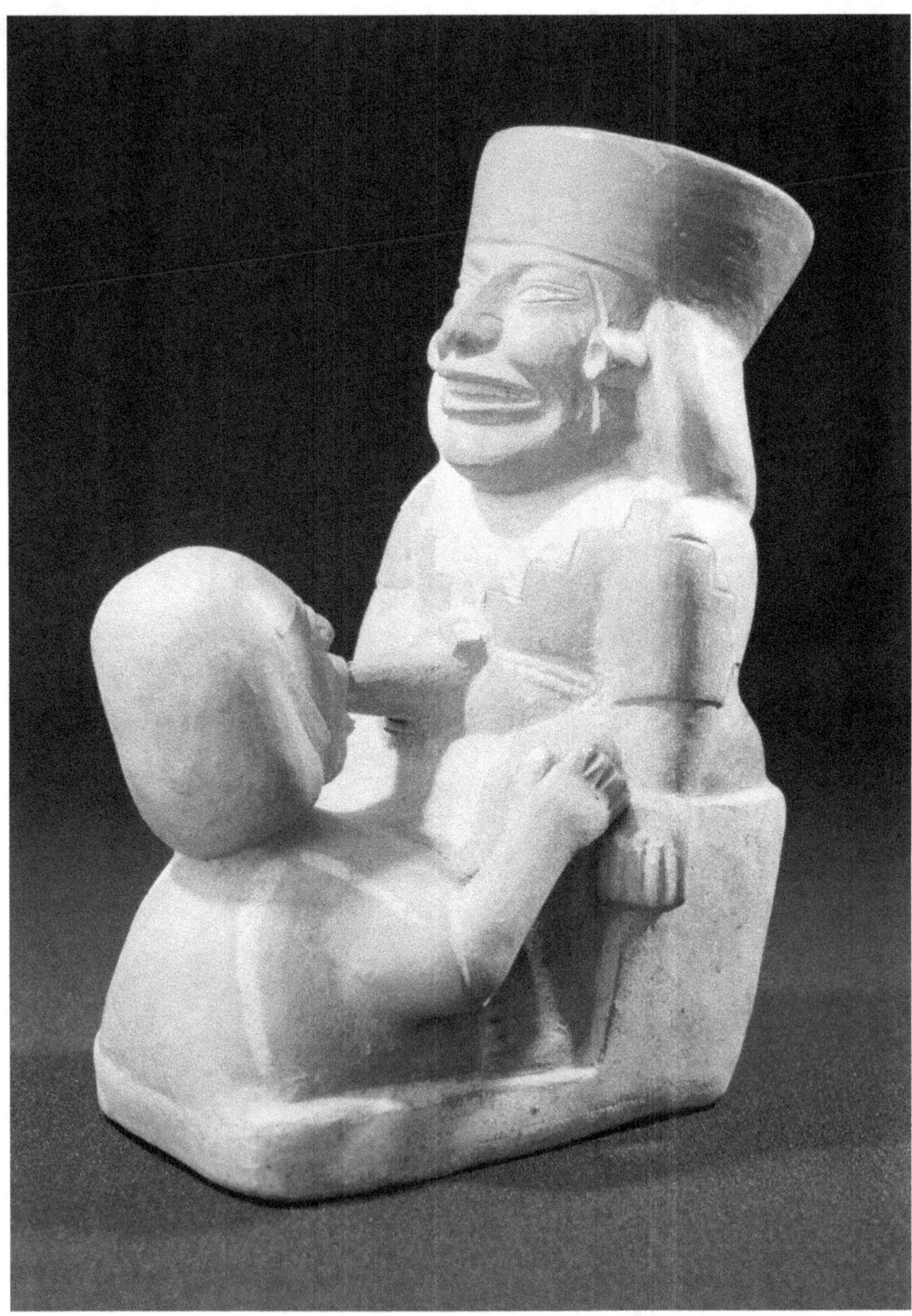

*Erotic Moche sculpture in the shape of a vase found at an archaeological site in Peru. Erotic sculptures like this were usually used in fertility rites by the Moche, a pre-Hispanic people that lived in coastal river valleys in northern Peru, whose civilization reached its height in the period from 100-700 AD. **Photo:** Pasquale Sorrentino / Science Photo Library*

"Glimpses of the Long History of Abortion"

"*Homo sapiens* evolved to be a slowing breeding animal. Prehistoric societies, like the few preliterate societies that remain, probably had total fertility rates of 4 to 6. Approximately half the children who were born died before they could reproduce, and population grew slowly. Puberty was in the upper teens, babies were breastfed for 3–4 years, and pregnancies were therefore naturally spaced by long intervals of amenorrhea. With the first urban civilizations and settled agriculture, puberty began at an earlier age and breastfeeding was often shortened or supplementary food introduced earlier than in hunter-gatherer societies. Fertility went up. In the modern world, if a couple initiates sexual intercourse when the woman is 20 years old or younger and continues at least until her menopause, without artificially limiting fertility, she can expect to conceive and carry to term an average of 10 live-born children.[1] Sooner or later, all human societies have to adopt restraints on family size."

"Ways to Abort in Antiquity-Medieval Times"

- withdrawal of the penis before ejaculation, aka coitus interruptus (Genesis 38:7 to 10)

- threshing inside and winnowing outside (Talmud)

- Strenuous labor

- climbing

- paddling

- weightlifting, or diving

- the use of irritant leaves

- fasting

- bloodletting

[1]Potts, M, Campbell, M, *Glob. libr. women's med.,* *(ISSN: 1756-2228)* 2009; DOI 10.3843/GLOWM.10376

- pouring hot water onto the abdomen, and lying on a heated coconut shell

- battery

- exercise

- tightening the girdle

- abortifacient medicines

- honey, pepper, alum, or lactic acid as pessaries and barriers

- vaginal pessaries from the alkaline dung of animals, such as crocodiles, elephants, or mice

- anal heterosexual intercourse

- https://www.gq-magazine.co.uk/article/a-history-of-anal-sex

- an herb called silphion (from North Africa)

- Embryotomy (removal of foetus with forceps)

- "If the semen has become lodged, there is no help for it but that she insert into her womb a probe or stick cut into the shape of a probe, especially good being the root of the mallow. One end of the probe should be made fast to the thigh with a thread that it may go no further. Leave it there all night, often all day as well… Some people screw paper up tight into the shape of a probe and after binding it securely with silk smear over it ginger dissolved in water….In 1958–1959, archaeologists excavating the skeleton of a young woman (20–25 years old) from a Gallo-Roman site in The Netherlands found a bone stylet 105 mm long in the pelvis. The grave was interpreted as that of a woman who died as the result of an attempt to induce a mechanical abortion."

- "Massage abortion is a technology that has been described in Burma, Thailand, Malaysia, the Philippines, and Indonesia. The procedure is usually attempted when the woman is 12–20 weeks pregnant. She lies on her back with her knees drawn up and the traditional birth attendant attempts to fix the uterus and then presses as hard as possible with her fingers, the heel of her bare foot, or even the wood pestle used to grind rice."

"Woman as Threefold Murderess"

The earliest insight into fertility regulation at the personal level dates back to the 13th century. The Cathar (or Albigensian) sect celebrated the sacrament shortly before death (the *perfecti*, or *heretication*, hence the word heretic). The Albigensians were persecuted mercilessly. Among the last remnants of the sect was a group in the Pyrenean village of Montaillou. Between 1318 and 1325, the local bishop, an obsessive man who later became Pope of Avignon, had recorded the confessions of suspected heretics verbatim to uncover incriminating evidence. The local priest, Pierre Clergue, had a particularly active sex life. One mistress, Beatrice, asked him,

"What shall I do if I become pregnant by you? I shall be ashamed and lost." "I have a certain herb," answered the priest. "If a man wears it when he mingles his body with that of a woman he cannot engender, nor she conceive." "What sort of herb? Is it the one the cowherds hang over a cauldron of milk in which they have put some rennet to stop the milk from curdling?"

The woman was referring to a theme in sympathetic magic that can be traced back to Dioscorides. Certainly, the sexually active society of Montaillou seemed to have exercised some check on fertility. Perhaps coitus interruptus was used. Most women had four or five children. (Beatrice had four children by her husband but none by Pierre.)

Some idea of medieval attitudes toward contraception can be obtained from the Penitentials—the religious compilations used by many priests as a framework for their work in the confessional. Sexual sin exceeded all others in the Penitentials. Noonan[2] has categorized the sexual content of Penitentials from the 6th to 11th centuries. A nocturnal ejaculation warranted 7 days' fasting, while contraception, fellatio, and anal intercourse attracted penances from 3–15 years. Religious records are supplemented by civil cases from 14th and 15th century Venice. Men guilty of homosexual anal intercourse were being burned alive between the Columns of Justice in St. Mark's Square. But anal intercourse in marriage was also sometimes prosecuted with exile for a few

---

[2] Potts, M, Campbell, M, *Glob. libr. women's med., (ISSN: 1756-2228)* 2009; DOI 10.3843/ GLOWM.10376

years. Ruggiero[3] concluded anal intercourse was a form of birth control that was practiced by some people at every social level, from nobility to humble fishermen. In the Penitentials, the punishment for abortion was sometimes less than that for contraception and was similar to that for coitus interruptus, although St. Jerome was particularly uncharitable in describing women who died from attempting an abortion as a "threefold murderess: as suicides, as adulteress to their heavenly bridegroom Christ and as murderess of their still unborn child."

"Ways to Abort or Prevent Pregnancy, 19th century onward"

- clitoridectomy

- oophorectomy

- masturbation

- extended lactation as a fertility control because of the suppression of ovulation

- very low coital frequencies

- coitus interruptus

- "dry cupping" the uterus, i.e. vacuum aspiration

- spermicides

- condoms

- Madame Drunette's Lunar Pills

- Dr. Peter's French Renovating Pills

- Dr. Monroe's French Periodical Pills

- Dr. Melveau's Portuguese Female Pills

- Emmenagogues, euphemism for eliminating an unwanted pregnancy.

---

[3]Potts, M, Campbell, M, *Glob. libr. women's med., (ISSN: 1756-2228)* 2009; DOI 10.3843/ GLOWM.10376

"An abortion practice in a Welsh mining community in the 1920s"

- the small, thin candles meant for lighting to the Virgin and would be pushed up through the cervix (Dr. Evelyne Fisher qtd. in Potts).

"Plants used as abortifacients and emmenagogues by Spanish New Mexicans"

G A Conway, J C Slocumb

- cotton root bark (Gossypium sp.), inmortal ((Asclepias capricornu Woodson), poleo chino (Hedeoma oblongifolia (Gray) Heller), rue Ruta graveolens L.), wormseed (Chenopodium ambrosioides L.), and three species of Artemesia

- The most widely used plants are cotton root bark (Gossypium sp.), inmortal (Asclepias capricornu Woodson), wormseed (Chenopodium ambrosioides L.), poleo chino (Hedeoma oblongifolia), rue (Ruta graveolens L.), and 3 species of Aremesia. The cotton root bark, when used as an abortifacient, exhibits the lowest toxicity. Rue is used independently within different cultures but may exhibit toxic side effects when used as an abortifacient. The plants are used by 3 principal practitioners: 1) curanderos (healers), who tend to specialize in the care of certain diseases; 2) herbalists, who use many of the materials used in traditional medicine; and 3) brujos, who are sorcerers and witches. Other plants used are osha, chuchupate-lovage; ponso or tanse-tansy; poleo-spearmint or pennyroyal mint; amolillo-wild licorice; dormilon-tall cone flower; malva; and, lanten-plantain. The least toxic abortifacients are species of Gossypium, Ruta, Ligusticum, Asclepias, and Rudbeckia.

- In 1844, Hancock and Goodyear in America discovered the vulcanization of rubber, and after about 1870, reasonable quality rubber condoms became widely available

- the diaphragm

- metal pessaries

- intrauterine devices (IUDs)

1959

contraceptive pill,
aka The Pill

YEA!!!

HOORAY!

HALLELUJAH!

For the first time in
history, women have sexual
reproductive freedom.
Legal. Cheap. Available.

APPENDIX II

Genre: Testimonies from women who've had multiple abortions

The anonymous accounts on the following pages have appeared online since 2015 at the Shout Your Abortion (SYA) website where this sentence, part of a mission statement, is posted:

> SYA envisions a world where abortion is free, de-stigmatized, and accessible in every community across the country.

I am sympathetic to women who decided to abort multiple times, though I've had the procedure once. I highlight here some of the accounts from women with multiple abortions.

My grief is not a political debate

by Anonymous, July 31, 2024

I've used the abortion pills three times. I needed these pills to save my life, and yet I still feel shame around it. My family doesn't know and they probably never will.

The first time I was young, in an emotionally abusive relationship, and just got out of the psych ward a few months earlier due to a suicide attempt. I was in no way fit or ready to raise a child. This was before I found out about my blood disorder which causes me to have blood clots and I very well could have lost my life, or the life of the baby, had I continued the pregnancy. My blood disorder causes late trimester miscarriages, still births, and even death while giving birth. It is possible to have a healthy pregnancy, but not without expensive blood thinner injections multiple times a day.

So the second time I took these pills, close to eight years later, I was in an extremely new, yet loving, relationship. The weight of things being so new, our financial situations, plus this fear of what could happen if we tried to carry out the pregnancy due to my blood disorder, lead us to decide to have an abortion.

The third time, a little over a year later, with the same partner, I fell pregnant again, despite being on birth control. This time, before we could decide what to do, I miscarried while at work. I took the abortion pills to ensure that all of the tissue of the fetus left my womb. I was devastated because it felt like my choice was ripped away from me.

I do not regret my abortions in the slightest, but I resent my country for turning my most intimate moments of grief into a political debate

I am still with this same partner, in a loving and stable relationship. And I have never yearned for a baby more than I do now. But the fear of not having access to life-saving health care such as abortion, or not having the option to abort a pregnancy if the baby ends up dying inside me, will probably forever keep me from trying to carry a child. I feel resentful and fearful of the path our country is going down regarding abortion access. And the grief just keeps piling on,

https://sya.im/share/60281 #ShoutYourAbortion

My Mom Had Five Abortions

by Mariah, September 6, 2024

My mom had me at 16. My dad was 21. They were never dating. He proposed when I was born. She refused, and he left. My mom got in to college, and when I wasn't with my grandparents, I was living with my very young mom and her college roommates. At home with my mom, I was constantly exposed to partying, drugs, random men, and people who should have never been around a young child.

After college, we moved to the projects. From the ages of 6 to 9, I was molested by a neighbor, who told me he would kill my mom if I told anyone. Eventually the abuse amounted to one instance of me being violently sexually assaulted. My mom was arrested in front of me for attacking the man who abused me, and I developed PTSD. Around this time, my mom got married to a man who was secretly physically and verbally abusing me — he would choke me, throw things at me, make up strange lies about me misbehaving, call me sexually derogatory names, and he conditioned me to be anorexic. I was a very messed up and very lonely little kid.

It took me a long time to come to terms with the fact that my mom was neglectful and abusive — and longer to understand that she was a kid and was also abused. When abortion access became all-but-illegal in Indiana, my mom broke down and told me that she had five abortions from the time I was born until my sister was born when I was 12, including an abortion of very much wanted identical twins shortly after I was hospitalized for being raped.

I am so grateful that my mom, with all of her problems, had the foresight, maturity, and resources to seek out abortions when she could not care for me like she should have. Had a new baby — let alone six new babies — come in to our family when I was younger, the abuse and neglect I was enduring would have deepened.

Abortion enabled me to save my own life. Abortion prevented more children from being neglected and abused. Abortion enabled my family to grow and heal. My mom and I are both lawyers now.

https://sya.im/share/55371 #ShoutYourAbortion

I had multiple abortions and don't regret them

by Debbie, July 12, 2022

As a teenager with ADHD I was dangerously impulsive, which sometimes meant unsafe sex. In the 80s no one really talked about abortions amongst my teenage peers, but we knew they were happening. When I found out I was pregnant the first time I was still in high school, and my only fear was finding a place to end the pregnancy without my parents finding out. Luckily we lived in a place where an underage teenager could get an abortion without parental consent. I found a Planned Parenthood in the Yellow Pages, made an appointment, went in, the clinic staff was kind, the nurse held my hand, and it was done. No regrets, just relief that I could still be a kid. And now, 35 years later, I have 2 adult children I was ready for, and I am so grateful that I could safely and legally terminate pregnancies I didn't want.

https://sya.im/share/41612 #ShoutYourAbortion

Even if conditions are "ideal"…

by Anonymous, February 28, 2022

I had my second abortion yesterday. I had my first abortion 8 months ago. I did not ever dream of being in this predicament, let alone twice within a year, but I'm thankful to live in a state where I'm not villainized for my choice and access is easy.

I had my second abortion yesterday. I had my first abortion 8 months ago.

I am a mother of three and my husband and I have a happy, loving marriage. Both of us have full-time careers and paid childcare is provided by my retired mother. We own a beautiful home and have a wonderful life.

Both times I knew I was pregnant pretty instantly (having 5 prior pregnancies, 3 children & 2 miscarriages). Both times my husband and I wavered the decision… but at almost 40, I felt done having children. Our youngest is only 15 months and a complete JOY — while a playmate for her would be nice, while we could easily afford another child… I just didn't want to. We didn't want to.

So I had a medical abortion, again, before I hit 5 weeks pregnant. While I am grieving… I am also so relieved and ready to get back to my life. Thank you for allowing me to share my story.

https://sya.im/share/6750 #ShoutYourAbortion

My 2nd of 2 Abortions

by Rachel, June 18, 2021

My second abortion story is very different from my first, in several ways. I was 34 this time around, not 20. I was at the beginning of a serious relationship, not at the end of a casual one. This time I was given the abortion pill series at a clinic instead of having a traditional "put to sleep" medical abortion.

I was 34 years old and 3 months into my first relationship in nearly 5 years when I found out I was pregnant. I was so over the moon over this fella. He was 7 years younger than me and had been my neighbor growing up, although we didn't know each other really due to our age difference. I had just moved home from AZ to CA and was renting my childhood home from my parents who had moved elsewhere. He was living several doors down after having moved back into his parents house with his young son who he has part time. We connected over hanging in the alley smoking cigarettes and me asking him to come over and help me occasionally with stuff around the house. We started dating and things moved quickly and intensely. Of course he started staying at my house almost immediately because why would he want to stay with his parents when I was right there and had more freedom?!

Well his family hated the idea of us right away. His sister wouldn't speak to me and his mom, who I had been friendly with all of a sudden turned cold. I of course was hoping to turn these feeling around, which I knew would not happen if I ended up pregnant 3 months into our relationship, which I did. Him having his son at such a young age was not something they loved, so me, this older woman getting pregnant would have gone over horribly. I found out on. Tuesday and made an appt on Wednesday to hit the clinic on that Sunday. I knew I wasn't having this child. At first I thought I wouldn't even tell my partner about it. How could this have even happened?!? I was 34 and had already terminated one pregnancy 14 years earlier. I knew better! We had gone away for a weekend in May and instead of being on my period I skipped my week of sugar pills and went directly to my next pack to avoid the bleed. I had done this many times with no problem, but this time it messed me up and I ended up preggo.

I was worried my partner would want me to have the baby, as he had told me he was "anti abortion" which is how him and his ex ended up with his son when he was 20. I thought that if I kept the child, it would ruin my chance of his family ever accepting me, but if I terminated it would ruin our chance of moving forward together. But how could I keep that secret?! I decided the day before going to the clinic I would tell him. I blurted it all out including my concerns about telling him. He told me he supported whatever I decided and was glad I didn't keep the secret.

Sunday he had his son, so I went to the clinic alone, which was fine. They took an ultrasound and almost had trouble finding the embryo, I was so newly pregnant. Thankfully they found it so that we could move forward and I didn't have to wait. The nurse gave me one pill which was to stop the cells from growing. I was sent home with another pill which I was to take within 36 hours that would begin the process of expelling the cells from my body. I went to work on Monday and then took Tuesday off so that I could take the 2nd pill Monday night. He was right by my side the whole time. Monday night was rough. Quite a bit of pain and lots of bleeding. Thankfully the pain didn't last more than several hours, but the bleeding lasted off and on for several months. That was the hardest part for me. I felt like it was different from my medical abortion 14 years earlier in that it was "easier" of a process, but it lasted much longer. 14 years earlier I bled for about a week after like a normal period. This went on and on… and because of that, even though I was on birth control again, I was so worried I would somehow ended up pregnant again, because my body and cycle hadn't normalized. There was no way I was having a 3rd abortion, but I knew by this point I didn't want to be a biological mom.

The boyfriend and I lived together for about another year and a half before we finally split up. Now that I am 40, I recognize that pregnancy for what it was. My last chance to have become a mom. I think about that one differently than my abortion at 20 years old, but I still have no regrets. I know I made the right choice for me and MY body and I'm thankful that I never became a mom due to outside or even internal pressure. Of course I wish that I had never gotten myself into either of those situations, but I'm so thankful that I had safe options that suited my needs as a woman and a human being who is in charge of her own body.

https://sya.im/share/4697 #ShoutYourAbortion

Two abortions, two experiences.

by Elle, May 18, 2021

I had my first abortion in my 20's. I struggled with my choice at that time because I wanted a second child, I was in a loving and healthy relationship with the father and it felt right. But I'd just returned to college and my partner was on his way to law school. I knew another child would change everything and make our lives so different from the path we were on. I made the choice so we all could have a future.

The procedure was painless. I went under general anesthesia for the whole thing. I had minimal bleeding and pain following. However, they gave me birth control pills that were not suited for me and they caused extreme depression. It took me months to come to terms with what I did because of this. But, with time, I was okay. I don't regret it.

My second was when I was in my mid-30's. I was with a new partner for only a few weeks. I believe I got pregnant our first time together. No one told me that Topamax can make birth control pills ineffective. Anyway, I was going through a bad divorce, trying to support my son on my own, and dating this new guy. There was NO WAY I was going to have this baby. There was absolutely no wavering. I made the appointment and went in asap. Unfortunately I couldn't get the abortion pill so I had to have the procedure done. I didn't have a ride so I had to be awake. They wouldn't give me pain meds either. It hurt a lot. Very intense pain during. But it was over quickly and the cramps weren't too bad after. I suffered a little depression afterwards but nothing like the first one.

Everyone should have access to abortion. My life would be so much worse if I had had to birth both children. My son would not have lived the life he lived. The partners involved would not have the lives they have now.

https://sya.im/share/6251 #ShoutYourAbortion

30yo, 3rd Abortion, Still Not Ready

by Shelby, December 9, 2021

I had my first abortion at 24, the second at 29, and the third at age 30. Each time has held an immensely different weight and context. I've been with the same person for the last 2. I thought I couldn't stand the shame of a third abortion. Or the heartache; constantly wondering when will I finally learn/be ready/grow up/find the right love and support? My partner told me he didn't want to be stuck with me forever when I told him I was considering (for the first time) keeping it. I knew I couldn't stand risking my life/mental health or anyone else's any further. And I couldn't settle on an unsupportive partner to be a coparent. I'm still not sure how I feel about my choices, but I'm glad I have one at all.

https://sya.im/share/6060 #ShoutYourAbortion

My 3 Abortions

by Shannon, June 28, 2024

I had my first abortion because I was very young. I had my second abortion because I had cancer & needed immediate treatment. I had my third abortion because I was not financially ready. Every single one is valid. Abortion is healthcare no matter what. I am not ashamed and never will be. I am proud of myself and was always confident in my decisions. Anyone who says "you've had too many abortions" would rather me be an extremely young mother, a poor mother, or a cancer ridden mother. I have 1 child and I need to be a healthy mother to her. Abortion saved my life.

https://sya.im/share/57668 #ShoutYourAbortion

3 choices made for specific reasons

by Sarah, April 5, 2023

It was 1979, the end of summer. I was living in a ski town and my boyfriend and I got pregnant. I was 19 soon to be 20. We both were in shock and he supported whatever choice I needed. My girlfriends surrounded me and drove me to the clinic. At that time it was very common. All my older friends, and my sister, had all been through it. It didn't feel great but the relief was grand, knowing at that age I was incompetent of raising anyone other than myself, barely!

In 1991, living in L.A., I was pregnant again from another (supportive of choice) boyfriend who I inherently knew was not my life partner. To this day I'm grateful for Planned Parenthood, their financial sliding scale, and the care I received.

In 1994 I met my "Life Partner" on a movie set. We traveled and worked physically enduring hours and I vowed I would never terminate another pregnancy. When I did become pregnant for my 3d time, it was too early in the relationship and I knew we could not sustain that pressure of bringing a child into the mix. We had broad goals we wanted achieve together.

This termination was physically and psychically the most painful procedure, unlike the others. That relationship did sustain for 23 years. We climbed mountains, made documentaries, kite surfed the Caribbean for a decade, among other adventures.

I never became pregnant again. I never have raised a child, and have had brief moments of remorse, but have been clear and respectful of those choices I got to make.

https://sya.im/share/56669 #ShoutYourAbortion

I've had 3 abortions and I'm done staying quiet about them

by Liz, September 11, 2021

I'm a 30 year old woman and I've had three abortions. All of them have been medically done via abortion pills. Seeing the news out of Texas this morning has really shaken me up. I did a lot of work to excavate the shame I had around my abortions after my 3rd one. I grew up in an evangelical church where abortion was a cardinal sin. I no longer have shame about my abortions, the only shame I feel today is the shame of staying quiet publicly about my experience and not writing in about my story sooner. My silence has been deafening. I am one of the lucky ones — I had access to abortion, I could afford them, and I knew I wouldn't have to face any extreme consequences for my abortions. Many people are not as lucky, and I realized today that my silence has contributed to the culture war we are facing where so many of us just stay quiet because the abortion continues to be so taboo. Our silence gives anti-choicers power. I am done giving them power.

https://sya.im/share/5219 #ShoutYourAbortion

My fourth abortion

by Anonymous, July 6, 2021

This will be my fourth abortion. From the same man I have been dating for 4 years. I'm not ready, and this has shown me I do not want any ties with this man. As I know now our relationship is toxic and he has told me many times I would be a horrible mother and he can't stand the sight of seeing me pregnant. Why would I want to keep this baby? And deal with him? No thanks. I am leaving him and I am starting over. Dear god grant me the strength and do not render me weak for this is a very tough decision.

https://sya.im/share/4783 #ShoutYourAbortion

Abortion number three, the hardest for me

by Anonymous, September 21, 2022

This was my third abortion. This was the only pregnancy I ever even considered going through with. The first two abortions were easy for me to know it would have never worked out with this man. I would have struggled. I didn't want to be a single mother. This time was different. I absolutely love my boyfriend. He is the love of my life and would do anything for me. When I read the positive pregnancy test, I had mixed emotions. Plan B didn't work. My boyfriend was scared but excited. He didn't think he could have children. I was scared. As the weeks progressed, I got more and more depressed. I've suffered from depression for most of my life. I thought about killing myself. I hated getting up in the morning. On top of that, I wasn't taking my meds. I would get panic attacks thinking I was harming the baby by taking my meds. We went to the first ultrasound, my boyfriend was ecstatic while I felt nothing. I was numb. I was going along with the motions of pregnancy, while absolutely hating myself. It took me until 11 weeks 3 days to get my surgical abortion. I wanted to so badly to make my boyfriend happy, as I know his dream is to have a family. I want a family also, but I want one when I can prepare for a child. I personally could not mentally handle an unplanned pregnancy. It still breaks my heart, but I know I made the right decision. My boyfriend still loves me and he understands why I did what I did. If there's no mama alive, there's no baby. I needed to save my life.

https://sya.im/share/55371 #ShoutYourAbortion

I had 4 Abortions

by X, December 9, 2021

I had 4. Accidents, abusive relationships and last with a guy who didn't want a baby and life as single mum with him in my life would have been too much for me. In the country I was born in there is a complete ban on abortions. At school we were shown images of aborted babies as a way of scaring us. The Catholic Church is very much against abortion. Where I live now I was met with respect and no judgement from the the health providers when I went to seek abortion.

I tried all kinds of contraception, some didn't work, some made me low in mood. I feel shame sometimes and its my secret what I've been through but I don't regret those decisions. I advocate and fight for women in my country to have the right to choose.

https://sya.im/share/5982 #ShoutYourAbortion

3 abortions

by Anonymous, January 15, 2021

I've had 2 abortions about to have my 3rd one tomorrow. I feel the most scared about this one because it is a surgical one where the other two were pills. Unfortunately the father of the baby and I didn't work out and on top of it I can't afford a baby nor do i have a stable place for the baby so I feel as though I am doing that baby a favor by not bringing it into a miserable unloving situation.

https://sya.im/share/4376 #ShoutYourAbortion

Third pregnancy, second abortion, and I am not ashamed

by IAS, October 18, 2021

Last week, I had my annual physical. While I was there, they took my blood and asked me the usual questions that they ask people who are assigned female at birth — when was your last period, and is there a possibility you could be pregnant? Last period was easy — September 9th. Was there a possibility I could be pregnant? Since no birth control is 100% effective, every month yes. I really didn't think I was, but my period was running later than it should — I had been chalking it up to severe stress, but figured it couldn't hurt to mention it to the doctor, who asked the nurse to tack on a test of my hCG levels to my bloodwork.

The doctor called me three days later, while I was sitting in my old childhood bedroom at my parents' house, to tell me that the blood test came back positive. It was not a difficult decision — I knew immediately that I would have another abortion.

I had had a very early miscarriage that would have been an abortion in May 2017 (5w1d), and an abortion in November 2018 (5w2d), just shy of three years prior to this, so I was upset that I was in this situation again, but I was strangely very calm — probably because I had been in this situation before, I knew what to do and I knew that the situation would be resolved fairly quickly. I count myself very lucky that I live somewhere where abortion access is readily available and I have the financial resources available to me that make abortion care financially accessible to me.

I was able to make an appointment for the very next day. I wound up doing the medication abortion this time around — I had a manual vacuum aspiration (MVA) procedure the first time, but they weren't able to complete the procedure this time (I was so early that they were having trouble dilating my cervix), so they gave me the pills instead. I took 1 tablet of Mifeprex (mifepristone) at the doctor's office, and they gave me the second set of pills (4 tablets of misoprostol) to take at home.

I'm honestly kicking myself a little for not doing the medication abortion the first time around — the reason I had done the MVA procedure the first time was because I had heard so many horror stories about how painful medication abortion can be, and I wanted to avoid that kind of prolonged agony if possible. However, I didn't know what I didn't know. In my experience, the medication abortion experience was infinitely less painful than the MVA procedure — it felt like nothing more than a bad period. In fact, I can think of periods I've had where I wasn't pregnant that were way more painful than this was. I took the second set of pills at around 1:30am; the cramping and bleeding started about eight hours later, around 9:30am, and I passed the pregnancy at around 1:30pm.

I immediately felt a rush of relief once I felt the pregnancy pass — there was no shame. No guilt. No "what have I done." Just pure, unadulterated relief.

We're told to be ashamed if we need even one abortion, never mind more than one. The fact is, IT IS NORMAL TO NEED MORE THAN ONE ABORTION. You and I are not the first nor the last people who will need more than one abortion.

The fact is, IT IS NORMAL TO NEED MORE THAN ONE ABORTION.

I have had two abortions, and I am not ashamed. I made the choices that were right for me and for my life, and I will do so all over again if I ever find myself pregnant again.

https://sya.im/share/5636 #ShoutYourAbortion

Happy mother = happy children

by Anonymous, November 20, 2020

I can honestly say that life has been really kind to me. I have a great career, an amazing husband, two beautiful young children and a house in a prestigious suburb. And yet I find myself at my doctor's clinic, asking for antidepressants. All because I terminated my third pregnancy at 6 weeks.

My rational side says that it was just some cells that I stopped from becoming a baby however when I see my children I just wonder what that little bean would have been like.

It has been 10 months since I had my surgical abortion and I still can't process my grief in a healthy manner. I used to run regularly but now the thought of running makes me feel selfish. Instead I have been over eating and gaining weight.

On my "due date" I had my youngest, who isn't even 2, in my bed with high temperature and I kept on thinking how could have I looked after her with a newborn. The reasons to terminate the pregnancy still remain but I still managed to have a panic attack at a family gathering. I told my mother and my mother in law that I had an abortion, expecting some kind of judgement but I was shocked to learn that they both had multiple abortions, after completing their family. We are Catholic women! Now when I am at church and see families with two children, I wonder if they had to terminate their pregnancies.

I was shocked to learn that they both had multiple abortions, after completing their family. We are Catholic women!

I am still processing this pain but have made an appointment to see a psychologist. Not for me but for my kids, they deserve a happy, healthy and active mother.

https://sya.im/share/4225 #ShoutYourAbortion

One kid four abortions

by Anonymous, November 17, 2020

When I was 18 I gave birth to my son Parker. Through the years it became challenging to raise my son, I did most of the parenting in my previous relationship. When Parker was two, I got pregnant again. I had this feeling that I wasn't ready for another baby. My boyfriend supported me, even though he did not want me to have an abortion. I thought long and hard about what my boyfriend felt, then decided to listen to what I wanted. It's your body and when it comes down to it, it's your life that will be affected more than your girlfriend's or boyfriend's. I never went to college or worked at a job before, I knew I wanted that in my future. During my years of college I got pregnant again and had another abortion. So far, I've had four abortions. There was some grief that came with it, but you have to weigh in the goods. I remind myself how happy my son is, and how much more I have to offer him. I'm happy where I'm at and as a single mother it's easier with one! I have no regrets at the end of the day, I simply believe that my choices made me have a content life.

https://sya.im/share/4209 #ShoutYourAbortion

I'm 23 and I've had 3 abortions already

by Anonymous, August 28, 2020

I had the first one on sept 22, 2018 (21 yrs old), the second on feb 2019 (22 yrs old) and the last one on oct 2019 (23 yrs old). They were at 8, 5 and 4 weeks respectively; all of them using Cytotec (misoprostol). It's illegal in my country to do this and had to buy them under the radar at a super expensive price but I could not be happier with my choice. I admit me and my bf have been irresponsible sexually but I'd rather be called that than have a kid that I will absolutely not want. It angers me to see abandoned or abused kids that could have been prevented if abortions were legal. It sucks to live in a 3rd world conservative af country but this movement gives me peace. **I regret nothing.**

https://sya.im/share/3972 #ShoutYourAbortion

Seven abortions, six Irish people in need, one protest, zero shame

by Anonymous, July 27, 2020

In a strict catholic high school ran by Irish nuns, I first came across abortion aged 12, in a religious education class where we were shown a horrific pro-life propaganda movie about abortions. The young female teacher cried and apologised and said she'd lose her job if she didn't show us it. One girl threw up.

I didn't give abortion much thought again until I was 17, and fell pregnant with my first real boyfriend. I opted for medical abortion and had a pretty horrible experience in a hospital room with a tiny tv and a toilet in the corner, and I shit, vomited and bled my way through the day, drifting in and out of consciousness and screaming in pain whilst my boyfriend looked on awkwardly as he watched daytime tv.

I was 23 the next time I fell pregnant, and I'm now 27 and have had a total of seven abortions. All of my abortions have been medical, however the law changed and medical abortions are now fine to be done at home, and my experiences have been so much less traumatic and much less painful than my first abortion when managing them at home.

I'm not proud of it, but I'm not certainly NOT ASHAMED.

I'm been refused contraception from my GP due to underlying health issues, and refused sterilisation because I'm too young and apparently "will change my mind on not wanting children". That's a whole separate issue. But I'm not trying to justify my abortions.

I see abortion as a perfectly legitimate medical procedure to remove a tiny cluster of cells from your body, similar to getting your appendix out, or a cyst removed.

I'm a huge advocate for abortions. The city I live in is a popular location for people from Northern Ireland (where abortion is illegal) to fly over cheaply to get an abortion here. In conjunction with a charity, I occasionally offer the people having abortions alone in an unfamiliar city a comfortable place to stay and experience medical abortions with dignity and privacy, alongside somebody who knows what they're going through on hand with pain relief and a cup of tea. I usually drive them back to the airport to fly home in the evening or the following morning, and have made a friend for life.

I've also campaigned for abortion to be legalised in other countries, and on International Womens Day 2019, joined a huge protest in Buenos Aires for Aborto Legal in Argentina.

I have a pretty good job now, a stable life, a beautiful dog, and I don't want children ever. And I'm still with that very first boyfriend from high school. Will I get another abortion? I really hope not. But I am pro-choice in every way of the word, no exceptions, no limits. So let's remove the stigma, remove the shame, and start talking about our abortions.

https://sya.im/share/3921 #ShoutYourAbortion

Abortions in my teens, 20's, 30's and at 40.

by Anonymous, December 3, 2019

When I was 16, I became pregnant.

I had been abused by a man in his 20's since I was 14. When I told my father I was pregnant, he made all of the arrangements, and told me not to tell my mother, and I didn't.

After my abortion was complete, he told her, and she exploded. That effectively ended my ability to trust in my mother for guidance.

When I was in my 20's, I had several abortions. Most were due to sexual irresponsibility on my part, but I was responsible enough to know that I wouldn't be a fit parent.

In my 30's, I thought I wanted children. After 10 years of marriage, my husband and I faced infertility issues (the issues were his), and I became very obsessed with becoming pregnant. Eventually, I succeeded in conceiving, only to discover that the actual idea of having children terrified me. I terminated.

So, here I am today…

I'm 41, and I'm 8 weeks +3 days pregnant. I feel that I am too old to be a good mother, and I have health issues as well. I hope to terminate this pregnancy soon.

Many, many people would condemn me for what I've shared here, and I would agree that I could have been more responsible when it came to birth control — but I navigated it alone. I could not rely on my mom for advice, and I haven't even told my doctor the actual number of abortions I've had, for fear of stigma.

I come from a background of abuse, shame, and mental illness. I wouldn't subject an innocent child to that… And giving my baby away would kill me, so here we are.

https://sya.im/share/3436 #ShoutYourAbortion

I've had 5 abortions.

by M, November 4, 2019

Abortion

In 2011, I was 18 years old and with my boyfriend for only 2 months when we found out we were pregnant. This first pregnancy was very different from the rest. I had just moved out of my house and finally claiming my independence. I never saw myself having an abortion. This boyfriend in particular was rather emotionally/mentally abusive, so when it came time to making a decision, he was very unstable… in the sense that he made it about him. I eventually decided for myself I should have an abortion because, "I didn't move out for this." (My home life was very unstable as well with my parents/family.) I was 10 weeks and had to get a surgical procedure. This was a bit traumatizing for me because the doctor (who is now fired due to so many of the same complaints) was making comments like, "you should have kept your legs closed", while he was sitting in between my legs, using the surgical tool, and I don't know if it was him, but the force behind him

& the tool he was using was rather painful. I was already crying my eyes out due to the emotional pressure at such a young age. Afterwards, I had wondered if every clinic was like this, or, if this was the way every abortion was carried out. I realized through the support I sought out that that was indeed a very different case in terms of having such a rude & disrespectful doctor. I found an article online about the doctor losing his job 3 years later for the trauma he caused on so many people.

Miscarriage

In late 2013, I experienced a miscarriage. (Same boyfriend) (yes, I was stuck in this abusive relationship)

Birth

In February of 2014, I became pregnant with the same boyfriend. We were technically broken up at this time, but just like in any toxic relationship, I was stuck in a loop with him. I knew I didn't want to be with him; he had put me through so much mental abuse, cheated on me, humiliated me in front of so many people & constantly talked down to me. Having his baby felt absurd. I went to a clinic to start the abortion process, but was required to see the ultrasound (every state law is different on this, I believe) & when I saw her, I just knew. I didn't feel this feeling the first pregnancy. She was just a little gummy bear looking thing but the size of a rice grain when I saw her on the screen, seemingly waving at me from my own womb. She was so active already, moving around in there like she had no limits. The ultrasound tech laughed and said, "look baby is waving at you!" I entered the clinic depressed & when I walked out, I was talking to her, apolo-gizing & promising her a better life despite there being no real proof of stability at the moment. I was even living out of my car, technically, when I found out. I went to get prenatal vitamins immediately after & vaginally delivered the daughter of my dreams November of 2014.

Abortion

In January of 2017, I was back & forth with my daughter's father. I wanted a normal family, I wanted us all to have the last name or whatever, but I also truly just wanted to be respected & loved for me. I couldn't have both when it came to him. I was very depressed & very broke. He wasn't on child support due to his threats against me if I filed. We hooked up in the backseat of his car one night after I tried to have a heart to heart with him & he took complete advantage of the situation, (he didn't ask me if he could do this; he didn't pull out) I became pregnant after this one encounter with him, but this time, didn't tell him. A friend helped me get an abortion almost as soon as I found out. I was 6 weeks. This would be the last time I tried with him.

Abortion

Late December of 2017, I was finally moved away from the city my abuser was in, and managed to get my own little place in a small town. I got pregnant by my best friend. He was with me through all of it. We decided to take it further & he moved from the city to be with me. We actually had a pretty decent situation, I finally had my own place. Unfortunately, he had growing trust issues with me due to my daughters father, and him wanting to move back to the city. (Not everybody is cut out for the country.) I simply loved him, but he questioned me every single day and would pack his bags after every fight. We were good for the first few months, then once we got settled in, he was so insecure. He'd start an argument, I'd give him the same answer, he'd disappear outside for an hour, then his mom would call me telling me we needed to break up because she, "hated seeing her son like this". He was always going through my phone & would get mad about things from years prior when we weren't even an item yet. I didn't realize this was toxic because we had so much history. I fought for it so hard because I finally had stability & just wanted a simple life. When I look back on it, I feel like we should have never become more than just best friends, and the more simple option back then would have just to let him go when he wanted to. When I became pregnant with him, I was burnt out & was starting to feel actual chest pains from how much stress the relationship was causing me. He was so flighty and was becoming unfaithful in the process, confiding in his ex & other girls about his insecurities. By this point, I was done and asked him to leave, but he wallowed for 3 extra months in my house. My friend helped me with the payment, & I aborted at 6 weeks. My sister knew about this one & helped me get to & from a clinic since the nearest one, with the closest available appointment to the town I was living in was 4 hours away. It was all in between the holidays. January 1, 2018 was a different kind of new year for me as the bleeding started on this day. It would be 3 months after this that he would finally move out, after I called his parents to pick him up from my house.

Abortion

In December of 2018, I got pregnant with my current boyfriend. A few months prior, in August, my little place I was becoming stable in with just me & my daughter, had been invaded. We were robbed & my camera equipment was stolen, taking away most of my livelihood. I met my boyfriend a couple weeks after that event & it felt like love at first sight. We were only dating a few months & we were long distance. I was staying at my parents house now, having moved out after the home invasion. We barely knew each other. It was my first relationship where we weren't friends first. He came to visit over the holidays, that being our only second time hanging out & I became pregnant. We both immediately knew we couldn't be pregnant. He traveled a lot & is very passionate about it — I was the most depressed I had ever been, despite being in a new relationship. We aborted as soon as we could at 6 weeks, almost barely; the medical assistant told me it may be too early to take the abortion pill. It was successful. I had a very dark couple months after that though, the home-invasion still affected me deeply for a long time. I hated the distance between us. I had also felt low for it having been my FOURTH abortion. I don't know anyone who has had an abortion, it's not something I talk to people about. I kept all of these experiences to myself until now.

Abortion

It is now October of 2019, and I am aborting at 9 weeks with my current boyfriend. I moved in with his family for the chance of opportunities in a big city, with hopes of making money at a higher minimum wage, so I could get a new camera, back in May of this year. (Same bf as last abortion) When we first found out we were pregnant this time, we were actually both excited… Making this the worst abortion yet. I hate knowing we waited this long. Due to my hormones, discomfort and insecurities, we started to fight a lot. I was throwing up constantly and having to tip-toe in his parents house; turning the shower on to mask the sounds of vomiting. It's already uncomfortable to have to throw up constantly, sometimes 4–5x a day, it's even more unbearable to have to hide it. I wanted to give my daughter a sibling. But after just 1–2 weeks of me being pregnant, he opted for aborting it. We have little money and his parents were letting us stay there for free so we could save money. Him wanting to abort after being so excited at first didn't sit well with me & I fell into survival mode. I felt as if he were being sketchy about a girl he started working with & when I confronted him about it, he said he didn't want to have a baby with someone who was ready to leave him. I needed to have a backbone for my daughter. In my spirit, I wanted to tell him we'd be okay, I wanted to trust that he was not my exes, but because I am who I am, I felt HE should be the one to tell ME that… I felt exhausted having to fight for my life all these years & I needed true support.

I am a pretty spiritual person, I personally do believe in God, so this whole time, I am praying for forgiveness & for strength to be my own person. I hated that I was excited at first & now had to make this decision. I started to resent my bf a little bit because of this & felt repulsed by his indecisiveness. I committed to aborting it, though feeling 50/50 about it, I knew I needed to come to a decision because he couldn't & that my independence was fleeting from all the compromising and trust I was putting into him. It'd be easier to just not be pregnant. It's been 6 months of me living here in this city, and I have not been able to find a job so I have recently decided to go back home, where at least I can afford to work & live with my almost 5 year old, and regroup myself, to reclaim my power yet again, but in a way that would let me know I have control of my life. I am 26 years old and I know what I'm capable of. I feel it is time to focus on my career.

I asked myself if I could do this by myself, have the child regardless if my boyfriend moved with me or not, but I added in everything else (his family, how they'd react, my current heart/lung condition due to stress/ my exes & always holding my breath, my financial state, knowing I needed to go back to school, my baby-daddy drama…) The solid difference between this abortion & the rest, is that I asked for birth control after I took the medicine. Also, this abortion was completely covered by an emergency insurance provided in this state, saving me nearly $575, which made me feel a little bit more as ease, the financial part of this experience from the state covering it, made me feel supported & like I wasn't doing something wrong to myself. This time was tough, but I learned a lot. While although some people can walk away from an abortion without looking back, this one specifically is taking some time to forgive myself for knowing how excited I was when I found out. I even told me sister as soon as I took the pregnancy test. I didn't want to lie to her, so it was another challenge having to tell her all of this. I'm very grateful my sister is as understanding & empowering as she is, her telling me it's not her body, or her choice.

Reading forums like this online & writing out my own story has helped me DEEPLY with my emotions and self-inflicted guilt toward the decisions I made. Thank you for the opportunity to share & thank you for listening.

https://sya.im/share/3349 #ShoutYourAbortion

Four abortions and another unwanted pregnancy

by Anonymous, July 1, 2024

I've had four abortions.

The first was in 2015 with my boyfriend at the time. I was 20 and nowhere near ready and neither was he. The second was three years after that. The third and fourth was with my husband. One happened because the person I was with did not listen to me when I said not to finish inside, and the others were sheer luck (or unluck) and Plan B not working.

The last one was just two months ago. I found out today that I am once again pregnant. I broke down.

I never imagined myself going through an abortion, much less five. I don't regret any of my previous ones but this one has hit me hard. I feel angry, embarrassed, sad and a little guilty. I wish this situation had never happened.

I know I'm still not ready (financially and mentally) to be a mother and neither is my husband.

I'm grateful to have the choice. I just wish I didn't have to take it.

I know I wont regret it; its just a tough situation regardless.

https://sya.im/share/54805 #ShoutYourAbortion

Both my grandmothers had abortions.

by a granddaughter, November 21, 2022

I am here to share my grandmothers (yes, both of their) abortion stories. One of them had two abortions at the age of nineteen and then at the age of twenty five. In between them she had my father. My other grandmother had an abortion at the age of forty five. She already had two children and simply did not want more. Neither one of my grandmas were traumatized in any way, and neither one of them had a worse life because of it. In fact, their lives are better. Two separate women, separate lives and families. I would not be here today without those abortions, and I'm grateful they both felt safe to tell me and others their stories.

https://sya.im/share/55894 #ShoutYourAbortion

Abortion number three, the hardest for me

by Anonymous, September 21, 2022

This was my third abortion. This was the only pregnancy I ever even considered going through with. The first two abortions were easy for me to know it would have never worked out with this man. I would have struggled. I didn't want to be a single mother. This time was different. I absolutely love my boyfriend. He is the love of my life and would do anything for me. When I read the positive pregnancy test, I had mixed emotions. Plan B didn't work. My boyfriend was scared but excited. He didn't think he could have children. I was scared. As the weeks progressed, I got more and more depressed. I've suffered from depression for most of my life. I thought about killing myself. I hated getting up in the morning. On top of that, I wasn't taking my meds. I would get panic attacks thinking I was harming the baby by taking my meds. We went to the first ultrasound, my boyfriend was ecstatic while I felt nothing. I was numb. I was going along with the motions of pregnancy, while absolutely hating myself. It took me until 11 weeks 3 days to get my surgical abortion. I wanted to so badly to make my boyfriend happy, as I know his dream is to have a family. I want a family also, but I want one when I can prepare for a child. I personally could not mentally handle an unplanned pregnancy. It still breaks my heart, but I know I made the right decision. My boyfriend still loves me and he understands why I did what I did. If there's no mama alive, there's no baby. I needed to save my life.

https://sya.im/share/55371 #ShoutYourAbortion

JUDY JUANITA was awarded the 2024 Reginald Lockett Lifetime Achievement Award by PEN Oakland. Her latest poetry collection *Gawdzilla* conflates the movie monster Godzilla with American imperialism, racism, and other ills plaguing American society. Her poetry collection, *Manhattan my ass, you're in Oakland*, won the American Book Award in 2021 from the Before Columbus Foundation. Her short story collection, *The High Price of Freeways*, won the Tartt Fiction Prize at the University of West Alabama [UWA], and was published by Livingston Press [UWA] in 2022. Her semi-autobiographical novel, *Virgin Soul*, is about a young woman who joins the Black Panther Party in the 60s (Viking, 2013). Her poem "Bling" was nominated for a Pushcart Prize in 2012. Her essay "The Gun as Performance Poem" was nominated for a Pushcart Prize in 2014. Her short story/novel excerpt "The Black House" was nominated for a Pushcart in 2016. Her 20+ plays have been produced in San Francisco, Oakland, Berkeley, L.A. and NYC, and are archived at the Jerome Lawrence and Robert E. Lee Theatre Research Institute at Ohio State University (OSU). "Theodicy," about two black men who accidentally fall into the river of death, was first runner-up in the Eileen Heckart Senior Drama Competition at OSU. Her collection of essays, *DeFacto Feminism: Essays Straight Outta Oakland* [EquiDistance Press, 2016], examines the intersectionality of race, gender, politics, economics and spirituality as experienced by a black activist and self-described "feminist foot soldier." She was a contributing editor for The Weekling, an online journal where many of the essays appeared. The collection was a distinguished finalist in OSU's 2016 Non/Fiction Collection Prize.

Her body of work, including books, plays, numerous drafts, recordings, articles and interviews, is archived at Duke University's John Hope Franklin Research Center for African and African-American Literature alongside the archives of other 60s activists from SNCC and with the archives of fellow SFSU activist and her ex-husband/labor leader Clarence Carl Thomas Jr.